Drink Moderately and Live Longer

Drink Moderately and Live Longer

Understanding the Good of Alcohol

Morris E. Chafetz, M.D.
and
Marion D. Chafetz

MADISON BOOKS
Lanham • New York • London

Originally published in hard cover as *Why Drinking Can Be Good for
You* by Stein and Day/Publishers.

Published by Scarborough House
4720 Boston Way
Lanham, Maryland 20706

3 Henrietta Street
London WC2E 8LU England

Distributed by National Book Network

Library of Congress Cataloging-in-Publication Data

Chafetz, Morris E.
Drink moderately and live longer : understanding the good of
alcohol / Morris E. Chafetz and Marion C. Chafetz.
p. cm.
Originally published: Why drinking can be good for you / Morris
Chafetz. Briarcliff Manor, N.Y. : Stein and Day, © 1976.
Includes index.
1. Alcohol—Health aspects. I. Chafetz, Marion C. II. Chafetz,
Morris E. Why drinking can be good for you. III. Title.
QP801.A3C46 1995 613'.3—dc20 95-94 CIP

ISBN 0-8128-8560-0 (pbk.: alk. paper)

 TM The paper used in this publication meets the minimum require-
ments of American National Standard for Information Sci-
ences—Permanence of Paper for Printed Library Materials, ANSI
Z39.48–1984.

To Marion

I am sad to know that
the flower cannot see its beauty
the sunset cannot realize its glory
the infant cannot sense its future
the steel cannot feel its strength
or the furnace know its warmth
but I exalt that moment when
exquisite beauty graced my eyes
roaring glory touched my presence
unlimited future soared my horizon
limitless strength steeled my character
lifewarmth filled my soul
what more is there to say

Contents

Acknowledgments   *ix*
Introduction   *1*

1 Carry Nation Had a Drinking Problem   *9*
2 A Brief History of Alcohol   *15*
3 The Best of Drinking   *25*
4 Persistent Notions   *31*
5 The Facts   *43*
6 Physical Effects   *51*
7 The Hangover   *59*
8 Alcohol and Your Health   *63*
9 Alcohol and Your Feelings   *73*
10 Alcohol and Drugs   *77*
11 You and Alcohol and People   *85*
12 Your Drinking Heritage   *91*
13 On the Job   *97*
14 Your Children   *103*
15 Drinking and Driving   *111*

16 Prevention   *117*

Epilogue   *123*
Index   *129*
About the Authors   *135*

Acknowledgments

Saying something positive about alcohol, as this book aims to do, is a risky business in these self-righteous times. Many of my colleagues who support my point of view would have their funding support placed in jeopardy if I were to name them.

However, I would like to publicly acknowledge the invaluable help of my assistant, Piers Bocock, who reorganized and outlined pertinent material from two of my previous books, and Marion Donovan Chafetz, my wife and coauthor, who updated the manuscript and refreshed the language. Her sensibility prevented me from taking myself too seriously in speaking to a serious subject. Her editorial skills are formidable, and I am fortunate to have such in-house talent. Scott McGlinchey worked with diligence and patience in typing draft after draft of the manuscript.

History is replete with accolades to the good of alcohol. The following are just a few of the many people who more or less share my position on alcohol, and whose perspectives strengthened my conviction as I dealt with an unpopular point of view: William

Shakespeare, Queen Victoria, A. E. Houseman, Sir Walter Scott, John Milton, Robert Burns, Alfred Lord Tennyson, Lord Byron, Samuel Butler, Charles Dickens, Thomas Jefferson, Oliver Wendell Holmes, Rudyard Kipling, Alexander Pope, Jesus Christ, Horace, Sappho, Socrates, Plato, Aristotle, and Winston Churchill. In addition, there is an abundance of salutary references to alcohol in the Bible.

I also want to thank Judith Kennedy of Little, Brown, who gave me permission to use parts of my previously published book, *Liquor the Servant of Man*, and my son, Marc, who put me in touch with Jed Lyons of Madison Books who suggested I rewrite *How Drinking Can Be Good For You*, now called *Drink Moderately and Live Longer*.

Introduction

Existence alone is not enough for us. Within whatever period we walk the earth, we seek to experience more than just the physiological functions of eating, sleeping, and reproducing. The range of our experience will depend on the chances we are willing to take. If we venture far, our risks increase—but so do the rewards. If we play it safe, our risks lessen—but so does the rewarding exposure to variety.

I do not presume to tell others how to live, nor do I want to impose my values on anyone, but I am bothered by what I view of society's mass marketing of safety consciousness and "social correctness" as clever manipulation of and hostility to social pleasures and indulgences.

True, such prestidigitation finds ready acceptance in a society whose values are steeped in the Puritan ethic of controlled emotion, eschewed spontaneity, and inhibited pleasure. Advocacy groups tell us about the risks of drinking alcohol; they tell us about the risks of smoking and being near a smoker; they tell us that driving causes forty thousand deaths each year.

Right now, in our lexicon, dietary fat has superseded cholesterol as the most feared household word, because fatty foods are suspected as a cause of cancer.

We constantly scrutinize our children's behavior and privacy, looking for signs of deviation from some mysterious healthy norm. Soon, I expect, someone will suggest that we avoid the bathroom because most home accidents happen there.

Over the four decades that I have dealt with alcohol and treated alcoholism, I have seen both the good and the bad of alcohol, as well as the promotion of fear tactics employed by self-appointed pseudo-scientific gadflies to disabuse alcohol and scare people about drinking.

Admonitions against alcohol date from antiquity. If you drink, the good people say you'll become an alcoholic, or a drunk. They also claim you will shorten your life, become illegitimately pregnant, damage your fetus, commit a crime, damage your brain, become an addict, smash up your car, or otherwise waste away. Alarmists warn of the evils that spirits, beer, and wine portend and advise drinkers to hide the bottle from their children. They pass special laws to govern its use, ban it from the mails, and control its advertising. Mind you, all this is deliberated, determined, and decided even as two-thirds of the adult population drink and enjoy alcohol.

My concern with society's emphasis on safety and propriety is its covert intent to suppress pleasure. Certainly if you fly the friendly skies or ski on fresh-fallen powder or smoke a Havana cigar or drink a frosty brew or enjoy sex, you risk the possibility of harm. It is true that you can be killed in a plane crash, and you can break a leg skiing. You can develop cancer, bronchitis, or a hacking cough from smoking, and you can drink yourself silly, stupid, and sick. The media daily spew out the ways sex can get you in trouble.

The fact is, though, such things don't really happen to the vast majority of people. Statistics show that most people who fly do not die in plane crashes, most skiers do not suffer injury, not all people who smoke develop cancer, most people who drink do not become drunk or alcoholic, and most who engage in sex do not get into trouble. Yet self-appointed alarmists driven by a minority of scared, unhappy people are successfully attempting to kill the pleasure for us all, and they continue, unopposed, to insinuate their messages of doom deep into our puritanical fabric. Their emphasis on alcohol is all negative.

I have worked in the field of alcoholism for forty years. It's neither a pleasant field nor an easy one. I know firsthand from my work that the destruction from alcoholism is great, the tragedy unbelievable, but let me make the following absolutely clear: alcohol *abuse* is a major public health problem; alcohol *use* is not.

This book addresses the average drinker, not the problem or addicted drinker. Nor is the reformer, who gets a narcoticlike rush in crusading against alcohol, in my audience either. Both the problem drinker and the reformer represent the extremes of the way people look at alcohol. The audience that this book addresses is the larger crowd, the middle ground: those who drink alcohol because they like it, and those who *think* they ought not; those who cure colds with it, and those who swear off because they *think* it's unhealthy; those who coat their stomachs with antacids beforehand, and those who drink milk or water afterward; those who take soda, and those who do not; those who have to get up twice in the night, and those who groan all day Sunday. If you are there, you are in the great majority of people.

Bookstores are drenched with alcohol literature full of terms like "hidden alcoholic," "problem drinker," "children of alcoholics," and "dependent personalities." The hook in these books is to make you question your drinking style by undermining your confidence. *Drink Moderately and Live Longer* is different from most of the purported "self-help" liquor literature, because I do not believe that most drinkers will end up in trouble with alcohol. This book offers the reader an opportunity to learn the fact that 90 to 95 percent of people who drink have no alcohol problems. This pattern of problem-free drinking is thousands of years old.

Precious little information has been presented to explain the historical failure of prohibitions. One can only conclude from the monumental number of failed prohibitions throughout history—from the Chinese monarch who, in 2285 B.C., sought to abolish the use of alcohol through banishment and execution, up to the Eighteenth Amendment of the U.S. Constitution which, in 1920, prohibited the manufacture and sale of alcohol—that people from ancient times to the present cannot be manipulated or forced to live by other people's standards.

The fact that people go on drinking as they have done for thousands of years convinces me that alcohol—or something pleasurable like it—would have had to exist. In recent years a few answers about why alcohol has endured have been unearthed by different people in different places; some are facts, some are conjectures, some opinions. They are gathered and submitted in this book. They show that alcohol came before civilization, and they helped to shape my opinion that civilization may not have evolved without it. Drinking alcohol is an integral part of human behavior in which humankind has indulged forever.

Among the many things said about alcohol, you will find statements such as "My grandfather drank like a fish all his life and lived to be one hundred and four." "My grandfather drank himself to death at forty-eight." "Make mine a double; I'm tired." "Make mine a double; I'm cold." "Make it light; I'm getting fat." "I wouldn't have done it if I hadn't been buzzed."

Surely there is no other human custom—save sex—which is buried in such a mass of myths and misconceptions. But I alert the reader that this book intends to weigh the evidence, for a change, on the good side of alcohol.

One word among the many used about drinking is "moderation." What exactly is moderation? Curiously, moderate drinking is beyond definition, yet everybody knows what it is. Immoderate drinking, on the other hand, means problem drinking or alcoholism. Some say that only a hairline separates the social or moderate drinker from the alcoholic. Don't you believe it—a grand canyon separates them.

The difference usually is described in the way the social drinker uses alcohol to heighten enjoyment, while the alcoholic uses it to escape reality. This, too, is not true. Drinking does not take the edge off reality for just the alcoholic, it does so for everyone. The crucial difference here lies in the definitions of reality.

To one person, reality is an everyday grind that can use a bit of brightening; to another, it is a self-destructive illness seeking oblivion. As you can see, much more than a hairline exists between the two. One thing is certain though: the social drinker is in the vast majority. If that were not true, there would hardly be a human race.

What, then, is alcohol all about? Why does a drink have the effect it does? What happens inside you when you take one, or ten? Why is one person a "two-fisted drinker" while another is a "two-drink person"? How about "swearing off"? Does food "kill the kick"? Does alcohol make you fat? What are the business advantages of drinking? What about teenage drinking, drinking and driving? What are the physical or psychological benefits of drinking? What effect does alcohol have on your sex life? How long has drinking been going on? Who started it?

The purpose of this book is to share with the reader the sum of my experiences about the good of alcohol in the face of so much negative news.

Chapter 1

Carry Nation Had a Drinking Problem

Carry Nation, that famous human symbol of Prohibition, had a morbid preoccupation with alcohol. She couldn't care for her daughter and couldn't live with her husband, because she was obsessed with "demon rum."

Is preoccupation a problem?

Winston Churchill, when reproached by his wife about his penchant for liquor, once responded, "Clemmie, I have taken more good from alcohol than alcohol has taken from me." It's a salutary reminder—especially now, when almost any action you take seems fraught with risk and peril. The water's undrinkable, the air is unbreathable, food causes cancer, or so you're told. You've got a lot to worry about.

The major concern of my professional life is the problem of alcohol abuse. I've spent much of my time trumpeting the fact that alcohol abuse is treatable and preventable, and that alcohol problems, by any measure, are one of the most serious problems the nation faces. And having said that, I still must agree with Sir Winston when he said that alcohol has done more good than harm. For when it is used responsibly it helps answer the very human need to communicate with others and to alter stark reality. And I'm not talking about immoderate drinking. For there is a safe way to drink, although it's not often talked about.

Americans delight in focusing on the negative side of things. It seems curious to me as a psychiatrist that my colleagues and I can define pathology very easily, but we can only describe normalcy lamely, i.e., as the absence of pathology. This circumstance is particularly true in the field of alcohol abuse and alcoholism.

We can talk about people who have serious problems with alcohol, but we're less prepared to speak to the issues of the vast majority of people who drink and, by and large, derive only the benefits of alcohol. There are books, learned papers, and popular articles by the score that define, describe, and offer solutions for the problems of alcohol abuse. And the intimidation of reformers is never subtle. They thunder against the evils of drink. Antialcohol advocates associate alcohol with illegal drugs to cast an illicit aura onto alcohol.

The word "drug" nowadays connotes a substance that is evil or bad. Aspirin and penicillin are drugs, as is another drug we copiously consume, caffeine, found in the most popular breakfast drink in the world, coffee. The Food and Drug Administration defines the word "drug" as "[anything that] is deemed to be for therapeutic or diagnostic use or to *affect the structure or function of the body*" [Emphasis added]. According to that definition, anything you eat, drink, or inhale can be classified as a drug.

The reason for this widespread, negative preoccupation about alcohol is that the majority of people let the alarmists dominate the public forum, and anyone who speaks well of alcohol has his or her motives questioned. Even moderate drinkers feel they can't admit to it without a wink and a grin. Almost no one was willing to say, simply, "Sometimes drinking can be good for you." Until now.

Even asking a question about drinking implies a "problem" with alcohol. The difficulty here is in perception; hence discussion of the *use* of alcohol does not automatically mean *abuse*. Problem drinking is not the same thing as social drinking, and when society is able to make this crucial distinction it will see fewer alcohol problems.

Arriving at this clear-eyed view, however, will not be easy. Study after study shows that people in the United States are uncomfortable about drinking. They are so ambivalent and guilt-ridden about anything that gives them feelings of pleasure that they need to knock its positive aspects: if it's good, it must be bad. Indeed, even many jokes on the subject are telltale, for jokes are usually a "safe" way to ventilate deeper worries and give social sanction to something people feel uptight or guilty about.

When you see someone out of control it threatens your own sense of control. And seeing an alcoholic makes you fearful that you, too, could become alcoholic. The likelihood of this happening threatens you, and makes you act in a moralistic, judgmental, and vindictive way toward people who are preoccupied with drinking.

And just how preoccupied are you? Do you spend time talking about drinking, thinking about it, worrying about it, and looking forward to it? When you look at the advertisements for alcohol, the message is loud and clear: after a hard day on the job you deserve that drink. Alcohol is portrayed not as a small pleasure but as a "special" reward. If the industry and advertisers were braver, they would portray alcohol as a mainstream item, as part of everyday life, instead of as something special.

Preoccupation itself is a problem. You don't have to drink to have the characteristics of an alcoholic. I think Carry Nation, that famous symbol of Prohibition, was an alcoholic—a nondrinking alcoholic. She couldn't take "care of her daughter and couldn't live with her husband, because she was so obsessed with 'demon rum.' "

On the other hand, Winston Churchill, by all reports, drank a lot, and some people would gladly drink as much if they could perform as he did. Sir Winston seems to have used alcohol in a way that amused and pleased him. Apparently it did not interfere with his functioning.

So it seems that problems with alcohol have as much to do with attitude as with amount. And there is a safe, scientifically defined amount that most people would do best to stay within.

There are, indeed, risks in drinking alcohol, and my years in the field have made me acutely aware of them. But anything that affects human beings has a potential for harm. Taken in excess, even oxygen and water, those essentials of life, can kill. Living itself is a risk, and I suspect the only sure way to be completely safe is to be dead (although some theologians may disagree).

With each passing birthday I become surer and surer of less and less. However, I am sure that I do not want to admonish, advise, control, or tell another human being how to live. I merely want to share some of the things I know with those who care to hear them. I want to dispel the myths and discuss the physical, psychological, historical, and cultural facts, as I understand them, about the good of alcohol.

You must make your own decision about drinking. You might decide not to drink at all. But if you choose to drink and you are armed with facts and free of guilt, you can, like Winston Churchill, take only the good from alcohol.

Chapter 2

A Brief History of Alcohol

Throughout history and around the world, alcohol has played an integral role in celebrations, worship, and fellowship.

In the beginning

C_2H_5OH is the chemist's symbol for ethyl alcohol, an anesthetic agent taken internally by human beings for thirty thousand years—and the practice shows no signs of stopping.

Historical references to alcohol appear in ancient Hebrew, on Babylonian tablets, and in Egyptian carvings showing the manufacture of wine. Wine was made in China before 2000 B.C., and archaeologists have unearthed the ruins of a huge 2,600-year-old winery at Gibeon, near Jerusalem.

The Phoenicians took "the vine that bears the wine" into ancient Greece in 600 B.C. Plato, Socrates, Aristotle, and Aeschylus were inspired by its spirit, and Sappho wrote songs about its mystical properties.

Wine and the god Dionysus went with the Greeks to civilize the Etruscans. The Romans established vine growing as an important agricultural pursuit, and after Caesar's conquest of Gaul it spread to western Europe.

Between A.D. 500 and 1400, Europe was the vine-growing center of the world. During this period, medieval Christians interested themselves in vine growing, and monasteries developed the refinements of viticulture.

But just as no one knows who discovered fire or who invented the wheel, no one knows what ancient ancestor forgot about a pot of fruit and later drank the fermented mash.

One fable relates alcohol to the creation of the world. Even then, the forces of good were contesting the forces of evil for possession of the earth. The good were victorious, but in the course of their victory some good gods died, and wherever they fell the soil sprouted vines. This battle raged all over the earth, spreading wide the distribution of the vine.

Persian folklore relates the accidental discovery of drink to love. A prince loved the grape to the point of autumn depression. To prevent his sadness, he stored his luscious grapes for future use. But time changed the flavor, and he was disappointed to find a strange substance. He labeled the stuff "poison," which made it instantly attractive to one of his wives who had lost his favor and wanted to kill herself. After one cup, her desire to die diminished. After another, she could not even recall her sadness. And after a few more, she had the courage to tell her husband of the discovery of the "delightful poison."

How ever alcohol came into existence, much has happened because of it. Some historians contend that it started the first stable community life. Early humankind was nomadic. Because it requires several years to develop a producing vineyard, anthropologists speculate that pursuit of the vine marked the change from a scattered human race to a settled one. When ancient Sumarians settled down to grow grain 4,000 years ago, it wasn't to make bread, but to make beer.

Not only is the discoverer of alcohol unknown to us, but the refined art of viticulture dates back too far for historical record. Ten generations after Adam, Noah is named in the Old Testament as the first to plant a vineyard. After the flood, Noah made his covenant with God and agreed to behave. The Bible records that he "began to be a husbandman, and he planted a vineyard."

The Koran ascribes the first planting to Mohammed's son Ham and notes that Satan was there, watering the ground with peacock blood, sprinkling the leaves with ape blood, drenching the green grapes with lion blood, and spraying the grapes with the blood of swine. The explanation: "The first glass makes a man animated, his vivacity great, his colors heightened. In this condition he is like a peacock. When the fumes of the liquor rise into his head, he is gay, leaps, and gambols like an ape. When drunkenness takes possession of him, he is like a furious lion.

When it is at its height he is like the swine; he falls and grovels on the ground, stretches himself out and goes to sleep." That was written a long time ago, but the picture can be chillingly familiar.

The use of alcohol in ritual services

By the end of the fifth century A.D., when Christianity was established by law as the religion of the Holy Roman Empire, vine culture had spread throughout Gaul, and the church was preaching and planting at the same time. In this way originated some of the most famous present-day vineyards in France. The clergy had the money and the wine and set the standards of drinking. The strongest wines were even called by the name "Theologicum."

In the Bible, Jesus tells his Apostles to drink wine in remembrance of his blood, and hence wine became an integral part of Christian communion rites.

The birth of straight alcohol

Straight alcohol could have been anticipated. The rec-ognition that there was some property in wine that made people feel better, vigorous, even younger, led to a search for the "spirit" of wine. To isolate this spirit required first heating the wine (while preventing the spirit's escape), and then cooling it to condensation. Thus, distillation was born.

Because the distilled product was more potent and more rapid in effect than the original wine form, it was first used as a medicine. Since the distilled product made people feel younger, it was called the water of life, i.e., aqua vitae. Even the word "whiskey" derives from "usique-breatha," the Irish-Gaelic equivalent of aqua vitae.

Alcohol's role in history

We've already mentioned how viticulture led nomadic tribes to settle down into societies. We have heard the stories of how alcohol's birth was interwoven with many different mythologies. We have also seen how alcohol played an important part in religion. Now let's look at its role in our own recent history.

As social evolution coursed along the path of history, alcohol gamboled alongside. At the end of the eighteenth century, the Industrial Revolution spewed forth peaceful rural folk to devouring factory slums. Crowded, filthy, and lonely, the exploited lower classes turned to cheap and potent alcohol for solace, while the upper classes sipped vintage wine in genteel fashion to lubricate social ease.

It was during this era of extremes that many cultivated uses of alcohol were refined. The aperitif came into being. During this period the arbiters of taste decided the manners of wine drinking. White wines should be drunk with light foods and the full-bodied reds with meat. The vineyards of France, Germany, Italy, and Spain became renowned for the special gustatory delights each provided, and the aura of status and culture was bestowed upon people who "knew" their wines. Although it was an age of strain, upheaval, and rough drink, the same period helped to refine the relaxed, stable tradition of good drinking for social benefit.

Alcohol and American history

The grapevine preceded Europeans to America. When Leif Ericson first visited the North American continent, he found vines already growing so luxuriantly that he called the area "Vinland" or "Wineland."

Twenty-six years after the first voyage of Columbus, Cortez, the Spanish conquistador of Mexico, ordered that vine growing become an industry of the New World. Cortez stipulated that certain holders of land grants must plant, each year for five years, a thousand vines for each one hundred Indians living on the land.

The Jesuit fathers carried Spanish colonization and vine growing up the western coast of Mexico into lower California, and their successors, the Franciscans, advanced into what is now the state of California. As each settlement or mission was established, vines were planted as one of the first steps in transforming a savage wilderness into a state of civilization.

Anyone who studies drinking behavior in the United States has to look at our Puritan forebears. Puritans were hardy folks who had fled what they believed was an irreligious, tyrannical, and besotted land; they were, by the very nature of their exploits, inbred with reform. They were indeed a brave, strong, and determined people, but they had less-noble qualities as well.

The Puritans gained a reputation for excessive devotion to drink. Their own writings indict them; their alibis and laws convict them. As a matter of fact, our Puritan forebears were openly ashamed of their drinking practices and blamed it on their hard-drinking Anglo-Saxon ancestry, their belief in the medicinal value of alcohol, and the hardships of frontier life. As soon as they had settled in, they began to import wines and malts; then came the vintners and brewers, and before long the Puritans were experimenting with their own vineyards. Hard cider and applejack crossed their path rather early, but it was Jamaican rum that really whetted their palates.

Rum, a heady emissary from the first European settlers in the West Indies, took a firm hold in the American colonies. Its success was instantaneous, and it spread with the force of wildfire. In short order, the manufacture of rum became New England's most profitable venture.

But as with other highly profitable endeavors, it

occurred at the bitter expense of others. The New England rum distillers succored the slave trade. African slaves were sold into bondage in the West Indies for slave-produced molasses needed to make New England rum. Rum founded fortunes, expanded commerce, enriched cities, played an important role in the American Revolution, and was used as currency. It is rum's association with the slave trade that is thought to have led to the expression used as an epithet against all alcohol, "demon rum."

Only the demand for a cheaper, more abundant liquor sounded the death knell for rum in the public's preference. Cheap American whiskey was being made in the border states among Irish-Scotch settlers to whom the making of whiskey was just another phase of farming. In time, the demand for homemade whiskey spread beyond the family circle, and the financial value of this sideline became apparent. Soon, the production of whiskey by farmers was so widespread that whiskey became the medium of exchange. The "hard" currency of that time was the strong sour-mash bourbon whiskey, which had taken the place of rum as the most popular drink in the United States.

The influence of the New World on drinking behavior was soon felt. Fragile frontiers in an uncultured, unchartered, uncivilized milieu resulted in the misuse of alcohol. Potent liquor was readily manufactured, abundant, and cheap. Distilled spirits were sought; fermented wines were neglected. Quick gulping took the place of relaxed drinking. This rush for immediate effect robbed the nation of the real purpose of drinking, and soon people became preoccupied with the problems of drinking, not the pleasures.

The focus on problems brings our brief history up to recent times. In the year 1820, some fifty years after we had gained our freedom from England, people began to worry that the per capita consumption of alcohol was too high (it was three times what it is today). Coincidentally, the country's concern about drinking paralleled a national concern with physical fitness, with its attendant quest for better health, better looks, and longer life. The battle cry against alcohol focused on lowering the per capita consumption. Ten states passed prohibitionary laws. The movement against alcohol and for healthy living lasted forty years and was abruptly displaced by the tragedy of the Civil War.

The next prohibition surfaced about 1890, accompanied by its consort, physical fitness and proper diet. The battle cry this time was the saloon. This effort resulted in the Eighteenth Amendment to the U.S. Constitution, which banned the manufacture and sale of alcohol. Again, the engine of Prohibition was derailed by another tragedy, the Great Depression.

The present wave of prohibition began in the early 1980s and continues to this day in the company of its steady consort, health and fitness. The battle cry this time is that alcohol causes society's problems: abuse, divorce, suicide, murder, drownings, and accidents that wouldn't happen without alcohol. In other words, the antialcohol folks implicate drinking alcohol as unhealthy and as the sole source of the nation's many serious health, social, and economic problems. A focus on the negative use of alcohol has historically increased the misuse of alcohol.

Perhaps the reader can now begin to understand why it's so difficult to say something good about alcohol. Fear of ridicule, political incorrectness, and a general unfriendly climate toward pleasure make people hesitant and afraid to speak up about the good of alcohol.

So much for history. Let us turn now to understanding alcohol; for if we understand, we will be unafraid to make intelligent choices.

Chapter 3

The Best of Drinking

Getting the pleasure from alcohol without the pain depends on knowing a number of things that contribute to your drinking response.

How alcohol works in the body

Alcohol is an anesthetic agent, not a stimulant. In moderate amounts it appears to stimulate because it inhibits the "new" part of the brain—the part that records new learning, judgment, and social controls—as well as those centers that control exhaustion and discomfort. A little alcohol makes you feel physically able and emotionally freer. Increasing amounts of alcohol, however, gradually put these brain centers to sleep. Then the "older" part of the brain—the center for our more primitive, less socialized impulses—begins to take over.

How much is the right amount?

Most people can enjoy the benefits of alcohol and avoid the pain if they drink no more than 1½ ounces of absolute alcohol *a day*. That would be three 1-ounce drinks of 100-proof whiskey (it should be drunk diluted), *or* four 8-ounce glasses of beer, *or* half a bottle of table wine. For more than a hundred years, researchers from all over the world independently defined this amount as safe. Today, however, bowing to "political correctness," researchers suggest a lower limit.

In an earlier quest for a safe drinking amount, Sir Francis Anstie, a British psychiatrist, made public Anstie's Law of Safe Drinking in 1862, which *also* stated that 1½ ounces of absolute alcohol a day was the upper limit of moderate drinking. (Sir Francis, a man ahead of his time, established the first women's medical school in Great Britain, and served as the school's first dean.)

Anstie's limit is an upper limit, a statistical average that cannot be applied to all individuals. For some people, even one drop of alcohol is a drop too much. Quantities may also vary depending on body weight and physical and psychological conditions.

How should you drink alcohol?

You should sip it slowly. Alcohol is a highly unusual foodstuff in that 20 percent is absorbed directly from the stomach into the bloodstream without having to go through any digestive processes. Gulping drinks produces a sudden, marked rise in the alcohol level of the blood, and hence in the brain. Even when subsequent drinks are taken slowly, you will tend to have an unusually strong reaction.

Besides sipping slowly, what else can you do to keep your system from overreacting to alcohol? You can do a couple of things: (1) Diluting the alcohol with plenty of ice slows the absorption into the bloodstream. (2) Eating, preferably protein and carbohydrates, before you drink helps to slow alcohol's invasion of the bloodstream and brain. An experienced drinker knows that, all things being equal, the same amount of alcohol taken with food in the stomach will provide a different, more pleasant outcome than alcohol gulped on an empty stomach.

When to drink

Alcohol is best for you when you choose the time, place, and circumstances of drinking. Obviously, if your plans include studying, driving, filling out a tax form, or engaging in other complex mental and physical activities, it scarcely seems appropriate to be under the influence of an anesthetic agent. If, on the other hand, you're going to share a meal or enjoy socializing in a relaxed way, then alcohol can be a terrific adjunct to the essential human experience of socializing.

The Chinese sip their alcohol, savoring each drop as a gift of God, and they drink to celebrate their mutual interdependence. Drunkenness and alcoholism are almost unknown in China. Having observed the practices of safe and healthy drinking in many parts of the world, I've learned that where alcohol is used in the Chinese style, people generally reap its gifts while avoiding its pain.

Where to drink

It's best to drink in a relaxed setting—in your own home, at a restaurant with friends, at any comfortable occasion where socializing is the main ingredient. Standing while drinking, for example, is not a relaxing way to drink, and certainly drinking alone is not a good idea. If I had to come up with an unhealthy drinking situation, it would be the American cocktail party.

Because the cocktail party is usually time-limited, I believe that people think they should either show up, exchange niceties, and leave, or stay and get drunk. The combination of standing, discomfort, xenophobia, and alcohol is not a wholesome mix. Another characteristic of the cocktail party is what I call the catharsis syndrome. Strangers will frequently pour out intimate details of their lives at cocktail parties. In my judgment, these outpourings are purgatives. Relative strangers sharing intimacies so freely in such circumstances are speaking to themselves, not relating to each other.

Know your drinking companions

Good drinking depends on good company. It's best not to drink when you're physically or emotionally upset, lonely, or in need of solace. Alcohol is no substitute for another person. It is true that alcohol's neat anesthetic effect will ease the pain of loneliness. It will free you to dream a little, to transcend the routine of reality. But what better safety measure for a flight into worlds splashed with color and enthusiasm than sharing the beauty and insight with at least one other person?

In other words, try not to drink alone.

It's best to drink with people who set expectations that are socially useful and not self-destructive. Look twice at the companions you choose to drink with, for they will play a part in the effect alcohol has on you. Regardless of where and how you drink, what you expect from alcohol is what you'll get. In addition, the expectations and tolerances of the people around you will help determine your own response— irrespective of amount. In other words, if you're part of a group that wants to act and feel drunk, even with small amounts, you'll act and feel drunk.

Americans drink to celebrate independence and individuality. The image they admire is that of the

Marlboro Man, an independent frontiersman who stands alone against threatening natural forces. Unfortunately, people try to express this ideal of ruggedness through their drinking. As a corollary, they focus on prowess, i.e., how much they can hold. Many Americans drink to prove something to themselves.

In a nutshell

The best drinking is responsible drinking—to be done as a part of, rather than as a reason for, an activity. To focus on drinking as an end in itself is the wrong way to go about it.

Responsible drinking includes making sure you have food in your stomach before you drink. It means sipping your drink slowly in a relaxed, comfortable setting in the company of other people. Drunkenness is a social taboo.

Pay attention to how you respond to alcohol when tense, tired, or upset. Ask yourself if you're uncomfortable around people who choose not to drink. How's your comfort level when *you* choose not to drink?

The cocktail of responsible drinking contains: a shot of self-respect combined with a dash of common sense poured over cubes of knowledge and stirred well with people.

Chapter 4

Persistent Notions

Purported facts about alcohol have passed into our folklore as truisms. Some, indeed, are verifiable, others should be consigned to the world of mythology.

Is alcohol an aphrodisiac?

Alcohol is an *indirect* aphrodisiac. That means when alcohol is taken in moderate amounts it relaxes your control centers and allows natural sexual inclinations to surface. Your inhibitions decrease, and you are freer to express yourself and your inner desires.

But freedom exacts its price. With more than moderate amounts of alcohol, desire persists but performance dies. You shouldn't be surprised. Sex requires sensitivity, and anesthesia deadens the senses. Heavy drinkers categorically have poor sex lives.

Is alcoholism hereditary?

Most studies confirm that alcoholism is learned, not inherited. Recent studies that point to a genetic cause are flawed, because the definition of alcoholism is flawed. There is no fixed set of symptoms that can be identified as the "disease of alcoholism," which passes down through the generations.

But alcoholism does run in families. Studies have shown that 70 percent of patients in alcohol clinics had significant people in their lives who had alcohol problems. Children of alcoholic parents have a greater than average risk of developing alcoholism *if* the wrong kinds of circumstances prevail. Caution, not fear, is indicated.

If your parents were alcoholic, the betting odds of potential alcoholism are higher for you than for the child of the moderate drinker. Risks and odds are generalities though, and they have no specific or individual significances. For example, when you flip a coin, the odds are 50–50 that it will come up heads. But if you flip it ten times and it comes up tails ten times, the odds are still no better than 50–50 on the eleventh flip.

Learned family behavior, however, gives us alternatives. What is learned can be unlearned. We can lower the risks. As a matter of fact, with caution and sensible moderate use, the children of alcoholics may be better off because they've been alerted to the danger signs. I have nothing against theorizing except when it becomes destructive to living. I see two dangers in the hereditary theory.

First, it reinforces the widespread and unjust sense of futility in caretakers who are trying to treat the alcoholic person. Second, it strengthens the self-fulfilling prophecy that if you drink, you'll become an alcoholic. If you're convinced that something will happen, chances are it will. Children raised to believe that their genes will propel them toward alcoholism have a good head start. Who among you would believe in a chance to change your destiny where heredity is involved?

Societies, when frustrated by a bewildering social and medical problem, look for a genetic connection to explain the problem, promise to isolate the aberrant gene, and dispel the problem forever. Alcoholism, in my opinion and experience, is not inevitable. It can be treated and prevented.

Do fewer women become alcoholics?

Alcohol problems do not discriminate against women; in fact, alcohol problems are increasing among women.

Many people believe that an alcoholic woman is more difficult to treat than an alcoholic man. This belief is based on the false notion that there is something different in women alcoholics that makes them sicker. This notion, however, is beginning to disappear as women assume a more equal role with men in society. Formerly, more women than men were reluctant to come out of the closet. Society believed that alcoholism was predominantly a male problem. Because society needed to hold onto its belief that masculine meant macho behavior and feminine meant ladylike behavior, women had to scream for help before anyone noticed.

Is there a cure for alcoholism?

The truth is that doctors cure very little. Surgeons excise the diseased parts, internists treat the symptoms, rheumatologists use drugs to relieve joint pains, etc. People are treated, not cured. Doctors don't cure diabetes, heart disease, colds, cancer, high blood pressure, or hundreds of other afflictions. If patients are lucky, doctors can make them hurt less and function better.

Alcoholic people can't be cured either, but they can be treated. One study showed a better than 70 percent recovery rate in the alcoholic population of government-supported clinics. Study after study reaffirms the finding that most alcoholic people can be successfully treated. The only untreatable part of alcoholism is society's fixed ideas and expectations about alcoholic people. In other words, a relapse in other conditions doesn't automatically mean the condition is untreatable. No matter how long the recovery period, a relapse in alcoholism is viewed as evidence of treatment failure.

People are prisoners of their own experience. Whatever people learn in observing a few alcoholic people, they apply to all alcoholic people. In my experience, I have never met an alcoholic person who, given an alternative, would choose to remain an alcoholic, and who, with tailored treatment, could not hurt less and function better.

Can a recovering alcoholic ever drink again?

Even in the best of all possible worlds, who would say yes? If you're a recovering alcoholic person you will have to choose whether to drink or not to drink. If you believe that a guarantee of abstinence means—in the classic sense—you'll never have an alcohol problem, guess again. The logic underlying Prohibition was the same: Remove alcohol and *poof!* no more alcohol problems in the nation. The world knows the fallacy of that logic.

I am not suggesting that alcoholic people try to drink again. I tell my patients, "After the misery you've gone through, why take the risk of finding out whether you can or cannot drink again? Alcohol is not a necessity of life."

That is sound advice, and many of you know of recovering alcoholic people who have taken one drink and relapsed. Besides anecdotal evidence, researchers have little to add to support a conclusion for one way or the other. Studies show that recovering alcoholics who abstain entirely during the recovery period are just as likely to relapse as those who take some alcohol during that period. Other countries do not place the same emphasis on abstinence as we do; yet they report respectable recovery rates.

The problem with the rigid rule against any alcohol *ever* for recovering alcoholics is that it scares off problem drinkers from seeking early diagnosis and treatment. Often, when people notice a difference about their drinking, they worry, "I'm going to be *forever* set apart as a nondrinker in a drinking society." That assumption becomes a deterrent to recovery.

I had no rules for a life-after-recovery plan for the patients I treated. They had to feel and function better according to *their* criteria. When I set my criteria for their recovery, the treatment was for me—not them.

Will association with heavy drinkers lead to a drinking problem?

Chameleons take on the color of their surroundings; people are not much different. If you associate with heavy drinkers, you increase your risk of becoming a heavy drinker. And many heavy drinkers, unless they change their drinking style, risk alcohol problems. Those of you with such associates should discuss with them your discomfort with the chemical barrier they raise between you. You should let them know you want a relationship with an individual, not a substance.

If the straight talk fails, there is no need to continue to punish yourself. Why risk developing a drinking problem for a nonrelationship? In all fairness, though, there are some heavy drinkers who do not create problems for themselves or others. However, should you pursue such a relationship, you might question your own rescue and omnipotent fantasies and check out your own needs. You might discover that you can relate best to people only when they aren't really there.

Some business and professional people have jobs that require frequent association with heavy drinkers. At long drinking sessions the trick here is to take one or two mixed drinks followed by *just* the mixer alone. For the rest of the evening, the rule is: nurse. Remember, when neither technique works, there's a lot of self-respect and dignity in politely refusing a drink.

Can a drink kill a hangover?

To kill a hangover with a drink is a lose-lose situation. There are two ways to a hangover: (1) Drinking in a tense, uncomfortable situation and being tense and overwrought (even at parties when drinking is part of the fun, there's tension), and (2) repeated heavy drinking.

In each case a shot of alcohol may bring temporary morning-after relief. In the first kind of hangover, the alcohol will block the messages of discomfort being sent to the brain to kill the misery. In the second kind, the victim is actually suffering early, mild drug-withdrawal symptoms: tremors, sweating, sensitivity to light and sound, headache. A shot of the withdrawn substance can relieve the symptoms.

In both cases you pay for this relief later, because you will have to stop sometime, and the longer you put it off, the more severe the withdrawal will be.

Do alcoholics have addictive personalities?

Researchers have failed to support the theory of an addictive personality. They can describe certain features that addicts have in common, but they also can describe other people with the same features who cannot be clinically labeled as addicted. They are unable to use these common features to predict who will, and will not, become addicted.

The clinical definition of addiction is the development of withdrawal symptoms upon ceasing to take a substance. However, many people are addicted to some thing: work or religion or play. If they are honest with themselves, they know that prolonged withdrawal of some routine tasks makes them uncomfortable.

Just as the alcoholic without alcohol will find a substitute, the addicted workaholic on vacation will work hard at play. Both have addictions, but the work-aholic isn't doomed to infamy by the label "addictive personality."

Can coating the stomach with milk prevent drunkenness?

It's not a bad practice to coat the stomach before you drink. Milk will protect a stomach about to receive alcohol. The fat in milk slows absorption, and the fluid acts as a dilutant. Drinkers who are careful enough to take this precaution will generally be careful when they drink. That is, unless they think that once they've lined the stomach, they can throw all caution to the wind and drink fast and hard without paying the piper.

Does alcohol kill brain cells and diminish intelligence?

Every second of your life from birth to death, body cells die and are replaced by new recruits. Brain cells die, too, and there is no methodologically sound study that conclusively shows that alcohol speeds up this natural process. If anything kills brain cells, it is likely to be lack of use.

The good news is found in studies that show intelligence—as measured by the ability to solve complicated abstract problems—increases with moderate amounts of alcohol. In one experiment, highly intelligent, well-trained people solved problems in symbolic logic better with two drinks. With four drinks, they were at their normal level of performance; with six, much below.

Are black coffee and cold showers the best ways to sober up?

There's no such thing as a free lunch. If you overdrink, you pay the price. There is no quick way (save a kidney dialysis machine) to clear your blood of alcohol except through the body's usual physical and chemical processes that break down the foods you consume. Alcohol is metabolized at the rate of three-fourths of an ounce of alcohol (about one average drink) per hour.

The caffeine in black coffee and the jolt of a cold shower may make you a wide-awake drunk—but drunk you'll remain. Alcohol's effects can be controlled only on the way in and afterwards by the inexorable process of metabolism. Only time and rest will help.

Does red wine make you sicker than white wine?

Too much of red or white wine will make you very sick. Although red wine is almost twice as acidic as white and contains more tannins, I do not believe a given amount of red wine will make you sicker than the same amount of white wine.

What about "Liquor after beer, never fear; beer after liquor, never sicker"?

When you drink beer first, the alcohol entering the bloodstream is diluted. You know that's safer. Beer also provides volume in the stomach, which slows the absorption of alcohol. So, you get dilution and delay—all to the good.

The other way around, when you drink liquor first (and I assume the liquor is taken straight, for if diluted the ditty is meaningless) you get a concentrated rush of alcohol in the bloodstream that is strengthened and heightened by the alcohol in the beer. I guess that's why a straight shot of whiskey with a beer chaser is called a boiler-maker—it's a drinking explosive.

Does alcohol promote kidney disease?

No, alcohol does not promote kidney disease. On the contrary, alcohol, with its strong affinity for fats, is little attracted to kidney tissue because of the low fat content of the organ. In Bright's disease, a serious kidney ailment, a monotonous low-protein, high-carbohydrate diet is often essential. In this instance, alcohol can make the patient's diet more attractive.

Does alcohol cause hardening of the arteries?

Pathologists tell us there is no evidence to incriminate alcohol in the inexorable process of narrowing arteries. Because of the vasodilating effects of alcohol and its strange attraction to fats, some researchers go so far as to say that alcohol forestalls rapid hardening of the arteries. Many studies find that alcohol forestalls hardening of the arteries and prevents occlusive strokes (the most prevalent kind).

Chapter 5

The Facts

Separating myth from fact is a hard job and a thankless task. Myths are comforting, but facts are unalterable, unsentimental, rigorous purveyors of the truth.

What is the pharmacological action of alcohol?

Pharmacologically, alcohol is a central nervous system depressant. It is in the class of barbiturates, sedatives, and general anesthetic agents. Alcohol has a dual effect. In small amounts its mild anesthetic effect on the brain results indirectly in the stimulation of certain functions. For example, your heartbeat increases, and you get an increased sense of energy.

Alcohol's immediate and most important effects are on the highest functions of the brain: thinking, learning, remembering, and judgment. The property that slows down the tense, driven part of the brain makes alcohol an important adjunct to socializing. But as the concentration of alcohol increases, mild depression intensifies, leading to sedation, narcosis, coma, and even death.

Pharmacologic examples of the release or excitement stage are manifested by exhilaration, talkativeness, mood changes, loss of social restraints, and emotional outbursts. At times the gait is unsteady, speech is slightly slurred, and certain fine discriminations are lost.

At high amounts, reflex responses, visual acuity, and alertness are diminished. In addition, visible drunkenness, heavily slurred speech, confused thinking, and weaving gait can be observed. At very high amounts, most people are anesthetized: difficult to arouse, incapable of voluntary action, and comatose.

Does body weight affect my drinking?

Yes, especially if your body weight contains more muscle tissue than fat tissue. Alcohol is not absorbed by fat and hence circulates longer in the blood. There is no hard-and-fast rule about how much a given individual can drink because so many factors contribute to a person's reaction to alcohol. The general rule of thumb is that a 180-pound man can safely drink 3 ounces of 80-proof liquor *or* 16 ounces of beer in two hours. For each 20 pounds up or down the scale, you add or subtract a half-ounce. Therefore, a 240-pound man could consume 4½ ounces of spirits in two hours, whereas the 140-pound man should have only 2 ounces in two hours.

Women, because of their smaller bone structure and muscle mass, should drink less than a man of equal weight.

Blood and brains, those tissues richest in water, receive the highest concentration of alcohol. The lowest concentrations are found in muscle and fat tissue.

Are alcohol calories the same as food calories?

The energy in alcohol calories is the same as that in other food calories, but alcohol's calories are different in other respects. First, alcohol provides no minerals or chemicals essential for good nutrition. These are empty calories (quick easy *zips*, but nothing more). Some beers and wines contain nutritious material, but I don't advocate using them to satisfy the nutritional needs of the body.

Second, alcohol calories can't be stored, so your body uses them first and stores food calories until needed. If you're trying to limit your caloric intake and are depending only on alcohol as the source of calories, you would develop unpleasant nutritional deficiency diseases.

Is alcohol a hunger suppressant?

In moderate amounts, alcohol enhances the appetite. Some doctors still prescribe it for patients who have lost their zest for eating.

But heavy amounts of alcohol tend to suppress the desire to eat. For example, when you need food, your body sends out hunger signals. But if your ability to respond to these signals is depressed, you're unlikely to make the effort to eat. The calories in alcohol make us feel satisfied only temporarily. And finally, a stomach lining irritated by alcohol won't want to receive food.

How fast does alcohol take effect?

Alcohol is a fast-acting agent. A tiny bit gets into the blood by inhalation as you drink, and up to 20 percent goes into the bloodstream from the stomach. Because it requires no digestive action, alcohol is distributed throughout the body in just minutes after it's swallowed.

Is it better to dilute drinks?

With spirits, absolutely and always, yes, it is better to dilute the drink, unless, of course, it is a brandy or other drink that should be drunk in its natural state. The concentration of alcohol in your bloodstream will reflect the concentration of alcohol in your glass. Spirits should be diluted with ice and plain water. Avoid carbonated mixers. The gas creates pressure that forces the liquid quickly through the walls of the capillaries in the stomach and into the bloodstream. Wine and beer need not be diluted since they provide alcohol in diluted form.

Does food "kill the kick"?

Food in the stomach slows the rate at which alcohol enters the intestine and bloodstream by mechanically covering the stomach wall. Lining the stomach impedes alcohol's access to capillaries (the quick way into the blood). Food also slows absorption by sponging up the alcohol and carrying it slowly through the digestive process. A slower rate of absorption allows the metabolic processes to adapt. In this way you won't overwhelm your system.

If alcohol is habit-forming, why aren't we all addicted?

If by habit-forming you mean physiological addiction, then alcohol can be habit-forming. However, you must drink a lot over a long period of time to get physiologically addicted to alcohol. Most people don't become addicted.

Contrary to common belief, taking addicting substances does not mean that you're almost immediately hooked. You have to work at getting addicted. Government reports tell of weekend users of heroin and cocaine who are *not* addicted. In my opinion, there is no such thing as an addicting drug. To be labeled as an addicting drug means that everyone who tries it would be hooked. I know of no such substance. As noted in Chapter 4, people can be addicted to many things and actions that are not substances.

Do a 12-ounce can of beer, an ounce of 100-proof rum, and 5 ounces of wine each contain the same amount of alcohol?

The form a drink comes in doesn't always tell you how much alcohol it contains. A 12-ounce can of beer has the same alcohol content as an ounce of 100-proof rum—the difference is in the volume.

A 5-ounce glass of table wine has the same amount of alcohol as a 12-ounce can of beer or a 1-ounce measure of 100-proof spirits. Five ounces of *fortified* wine (such as vermouth, sherry, or port) would contain 75 percent more alcohol than the 12-ounce can of beer or 1-ounce measure of spirits.

In vodka you can find great variation in potency—from 80-proof up to 150-proof. It's wise to know the alcohol content of what you drink. The alcohol content of spirits is kept high by federal law. The government's standards of identity require that a product labeled as gin, tequila, rum, bourbon, vodka, scotch, or rye, and so on, must be at least 80-proof. Those products with less than 80-proof must have the word *diluted* printed on the label in the same type size as the statement of class. This government oversight discourages manufacturers from marketing lower-proof products.

Is alcohol stronger in certain drinks?

The alcohol in whiskey is not stronger than the *same* amount of alcohol in wine or beer. The difference in effect depends on the rate at which the alcohol reaches the brain. The person who drinks whiskey straight usually drinks it in a few minutes, while the wine or beer drinker will take longer to consume the same amount of alcohol, because of dilution and volume. Even when the wine or beer drinker takes in more *actual* alcohol, the continuous oxidation and elimination of alcohol by the body over the longer time span results in a lower blood-alcohol concentration. Of course, well-diluted whiskey sipped slowly will have the same moderating effect as wine or beer.

What is denatured alcohol?

Denatured alcohol is ethyl alcohol which has been purposefully contaminated. Chemicals such as methyl alcohol, benzine, or pyridine are added to ethyl alcohol to make it smell and taste bad. Denatured alcohol is used to make commercial products from shellac to antifreeze. The alcohol is contaminated so employees won't drink it.

Is there a difference between rubbing alcohol and the alcohol I drink?

Rubbing alcohol is impotable alcohol and is used topically to help bring down a fever, make the bedridden more comfortable, and cleanse the skin.

The form of alcohol used is isopropyl, a by-product of the petroleum and natural gas industry. It tastes terrible and will make you very sick if you drink it.

What does being "high" mean? What does alcohol do to make me feel and act this way?

Being "high" is when both feet are on the ground, yet you're flying because you've consumed more alcohol than the body can metabolize at the steady rate of three-fourths of an ounce of absolute alcohol per hour. As alcohol dampens the higher brain centers affecting judgment, perception, and social controls, the deep brain centers take over. When this happens, your perceptions dim, and you move from familiar patterns to instinctual behavior. Familiar landmarks are lost. It's like flying a plane without a horizon indicator. You become discombobulated.

Chapter 6

Physical Effects

Alcohol can affect your weight, sex life, appearance, and reality.

Why do I gain weight when I stop drinking?

Some people drink because they have an unusual need for fluids (polydipsia). Other people have an uncommon need for oral stimulation. For both the social drinker and the alcoholic person, when alcohol is removed for any reason, substitutes are sought.

However, the vast majority of social drinkers do not gain weight when they stop drinking. But, not uncommonly, social drinkers will nosh on whatever's available while their companions are drinking. Abstaining social drinkers will pop more peanuts or other finger-type foods just to feel part of the group. These foods, especially nuts, have a high fat content.

Also, some social drinkers have emotional needs that are unrequited, and they've used alcohol in the

51

past to relieve momentary loneliness. Alcohol replaced the comfort and satisfaction of a relationship with another person. When social drinkers stop drinking, they should be cautious, discreet, and watchful.

On the other hand, the alcoholic person who stops drinking needs to deal with the pain of heavy-duty problems. The hunger for solace often leads to a large weight gain. Alcoholics Anonymous meetings operate with barrels of coffee (often with cream and sugar) and gallons of carbonated drinks, which supply not only liquid but calories.

It is a natural phenomenon to fill the loss of one thing with another.

Are some kinds of alcohol less fattening than others?

This is the kind of question that drives experts to drink—Evian. Their frustration lies in the lack of precision in calorie charts. Because people believe in the certainty of numbers, they think calorie charts are beyond reproach. They are not. I've rarely found two charts that use the same figures when they describe equivalent drinks.

An ounce of absolute alcohol generally provides 150 to 200 calories.

What about the "Drinking Man's Diet"?

If you want to lose weight, I'd suggest that you give up drinking while dieting. Even small amounts of alcohol can affect recent memory and judgment. Those of you like Oscar Wilde who can resist everything but temptation had best not challenge your resolve. It's hard enough to say a noble "No" when your determination is strong.

Moreover, alcohol in moderation stimulates the appetite. An appetite stimulant is counterproductive to weight loss. The "Drinking Man's Diet" tells you how to drink and lose weight. The only weight loss I've noticed associated with drinking is the emaciated look of Skid Row alcoholic people.

Do drinkers have better sex lives than nondrinkers?

Drinking is indeed a popular pastime, and some alcohol advertisers would like us to believe that drinkers have better sex lives than nondrinkers. Americans are inordinately preoccupied with achieving "better" sex. But the question to answer here is better than what?— the last one, the mythologized one, the advertised one, or the dreamed-about one? People still faithfully believe that a magic formula will make them relate better to each other, and "great" sex is thought to be the quintessence of interpersonal relations. As the French say, *joie d'amour* is delicate, sensitive, and shouldn't be rushed.

I believe that moderate drinkers, generally, have better sex lives than nondrinkers. In this instance I equate "better" with "freer." For example, by drinking alcohol you consent to relaxing your control. And since relaxation helps achieve the goal of better sex, I think moderate drinkers have better sex lives than nondrinkers.

What causes a beer belly?

Beer is a high-caloric drink, and the giant breweries acknowledge this by promoting light beers, hoping to appeal to weight watchers.

When you are in the prime of life, your chest is muscular and strong. Middle age begins when your chest, responding to gravity, shifts to your belly, and, like the migrating bird flying south, a roll of fat finds your middle. Presto! A beer belly. For those whose major recreational activity is sitting on a bar stool or lounging on a couch watching TV, be prepared for the fall of the Holy Roman Empire!

What causes a red nose?

One of the actions of alcohol is vasodilation—a dilating or opening of blood vessels. This action takes place when alcohol affects the brain centers that influence the structure of vessel walls.

When it's cold outside, your blood tends to pool up deep within your body to preserve heat. It's one of the reasons you turn bluish—the blood has essentially fled from the surface of your skin. That is why you feel warm from a drink when you are cold, and the very reason it would be unwise to drink a lot when exposed to frigid climes.

Capillaries, the tiniest of blood vessels, are most exposed in the nose, which is most exposed to the elements. Engorged, blood-rich capillaries exposed to cold or trauma often break, causing the nose to become red. A rosy proboscis is not an uncommon sight in frequent heavy drinkers, a la W. C. Fields. I suspect that Mother Nature—in her way of mocking us—lights up the noses of people who do not responsibly use or appreciate her gifts.

Why do I get thirsty when I drink?

Alcohol, acting like a diuretic, causes more than normal amounts of water to flow through the kidneys. Some people who experience this diuretic activity get a thirst. Still others who use alcohol externally as an astringent think drinking dries them out internally as well, and they, too, feel thirsty.

However, the thirst that comes with drinking is physiological and comes from an imbalance in the fluid level of the cells' membranes. Alcohol and its mineral content (especially sodium) causes fluids to diffuse into the spaces surrounding the cells' membranes. When the water balance shifts from the cell to intercellular space, you will feel thirsty. Thirst signals alert you to restore water levels to dilute the salts that affect electrolytic balance.

You won't feel thirsty if your drink is well diluted.

What happens to heavy drinkers when they stop drinking?

The desire for fluids knows no bounds when the heavy drinker stops drinking. This is not a passing phenomenon but a symptom of withdrawal, similar, but on a much larger scale, to that which happens to the social drinker.

Moderate drinking causes mild, nontraumatic water shifts in the body; prolonged heavy drinking causes more profound shifts. The shift of fluids from intracellular to intercellular spaces overwhelms the rebound action of osmosis. People who drink heavily are not as able, as moderate drinkers are, to notice this change.

Eating sweets is a well-known substitute for comfort, love, and affection. Besides attending to emotional needs, gorging on fluids and sweets gives the bladder and stomach a pleasurable sensation of fullness. A couple of psychiatric interpretations claim to explain this obvious phenomenon: it fills a need for love or it is an expression of self-loathing.

Sometimes I have a few drinks but I don't feel it. Why?

Sometimes it happens. And when it does, you might as well have saved your money. Human beings can have countless different responses to a given amount of alcohol. The effects of alcohol on social drinkers who are tense in a drinking situation and may not know it will reflect that tension. At another time the same social drinker may be upbeat and relaxed, and the alcohol will not have an impact. Still a third drinking episode may be just great, producing a wonderful feeling of happiness and enthusiasm. Such a response to alcohol is wonderful but delicate. There are times when the drinker aims for this delicate goal but becomes mildly tipsy.

So why does a given amount of alcohol sometimes not provide the effect you want? It might simply be a time when you've unconsciously set your will against letting anything affect you.

All things being equal, drinking with a good friend will produce one kind of effect, and drinking with your boss will produce a different effect. With your friend, you would probably feel free. With your boss, you'd be in control.

There are times when what we expect and what we get do not necessarily establish patterns. For these reasons, experienced social drinkers pay close attention to how an occasion's drinking is affecting them.

Why do I get the "bed spins" after drinking?

The merry-go-round effect is a hypotensive response due to alcohol's property as a vasodilator. There is a short period when the blood pressure rises after drinking, after which the vasodilating effect causes a mild drop in blood pressure. With or without alcohol, some people suffer postural hypotension—naturally low blood pressure, and it's quite likely that even a little alcohol will make them dizzy.

But when you drink and lie down, postural hypotension along with the vasodilating property of alcohol can give you the "bed spins."

Why do I get tipsy after three drinks, while my friend, who is short and skinny, needs ten to get tipsy?

Amount and size is one answer. Expectation and control is another.

You might be tipsy because you gulped three drinks in fifteen minutes on an empty stomach. Your short, skinny friend with food in his stomach may take thirty to forty-five minutes to finish a drink. Moreover, your friend may need to keep in tight control of himself so that nobody will talk about the guy who needs to down ten drinks.

Another answer addresses the phenomenon of tolerance: increasing amounts are required to produce a previous effect. We don't fully understand it, but we see it. The tolerance response manifests itself usually in people who are alcohol dependent.

We still have much to find out about the action of alcohol, but know one thing: Never envy a heavy drinker who does not seem to get tipsy. Alcoholism may be the next station on his train ride.

Chapter 7

The Hangover

Try as you might to drink sensibly, there'll come a day when you'll try to drink someone under the table, and you'll be struck with swift, just retribution—the hangover.

What is a hangover?

Unpleasant physical effects called hangovers very often follow the heavy use of alcohol. The physiological symptoms of a hangover are caused by fatigue. Heavy use of alcohol anesthetizes the signals that tell you your nerves and muscles are exhausted. You do not know you've pushed yourself beyond endurance, because the protective warning systems aren't functioning. Nausea, gastritis, headache, and anxiety are the rude awakenings of a disrupted bodily system.

Complications and specific discomforts are related to the type of food eaten, the type of alcohol drunk, and the congener content (natural additives in alcohol that add color, aroma, and flavor).

Why is a hangover?

A hangover is misery worn like a badge. Despite all the concoctions and advice to ease the suffering, and with the promise of untold riches for the person who conquers its blight, many Americans actually take pride in their hangovers. It's proof of a "big night."

Observe the ready tolerance shown to a person in the vise of a hangover: the knowing smile, the kidding remark, the complete acceptance of his or her state of misery.

I know of no easy familiarity with hangovers in such countries as China, Israel, Spain, Italy, or Lebanon. Interestingly, the countries that court hangovers are the countries with big or growing alcohol problems.

Societies that place alcohol in the proper perspective and use it sensibly have few drinking problems, and hangovers are rare. But in societies where heavy drinking is winked at, where getting drunk is sanctioned, where people are conflicted, ambivalent, and guilty about drinking, hangovers are pandemic. A lot of Americans are "uptight" drinkers. The following conditions should predispose anyone to a hangover: (1) Tense or uptight drinking, (2) conflict and guilt about drinking, (3) ignorance of the anesthetic effect of alcohol, and (4) foolishness about its use.

Can hangovers be avoided?

Mild, occasional hangovers cannot be avoided. With or without alcohol, you can experience hangover symptoms (headaches, shakiness, and so on) when you push yourself too far, and you fail to respond to the signals that tell you enough is enough. In this condition, even a drink or two may well overwhelm your warning system; pushing yourself further lays the groundwork for a huge hangover. In this instance alcohol is the facilitator rather than the cause.

How to treat a hangover

Since fatigue is the root cause of your hangover, rest is the best therapy. There is no way to put off your body's need for plenty of rest in order to recover. If your stomach is not upset, aspirin or other analgesics will lessen the aches, pains, and headaches common to hangovers. Stay away from alcohol—it only delays the moment of reckoning. It's a very good idea to practice abstinence for seventy-two hours for a mild hangover and a week to ten days for a severe hangover.

Clear fluids are helpful. Some advisers suggest whiffs of oxygen. Copious concoctions are recommended, but to my knowledge none can substitute for the most important thing the body needs: rest.

How to avoid a hangover

If you plan to drink a lot, you can protect yourself from the miseries of a hangover. A few simple steps will help: Eat some food before beginning to drink. Sip the first drink slowly for thirty to forty minutes. Sip well-diluted drinks while continuing to snack. Make sure you do all this in a relaxed setting. And, good luck.

If NASA can put a man on the moon, why hasn't someone invented a pill to cure the hangover?

I guess the awesomely sophisticated mechanical problems NASA solves to orbit the earth are still less complex and easier to resolve than dealing with the problems of the emotional responses of fear, guilt, ambivalence, and loneliness.

Hangover cures are unlikely to come until we cease being human and become mechanical.

Does switching drinks (e.g., gin to bourbon to whiskey) or do carbonated mixers affect my hangover?

Switching drinks does not cause hangovers. The culprit is in the concentration of alcohol, not the kind of drink. Some scientists contend that congeners reinforce and intensify hangovers.

Chapter 8

Alcohol and Your Health

Even one drink can have measurable physical effects on you. And for some conditions these effects can provide an unexpected medical benefit.

If I drink moderately, will I live longer?

Advances in modern medicine and changes in lifestyle behavior have added a generation more to your life. Statistics tell us that moderate drinkers live longer than ex-drinkers, heavy drinkers, and abstainers, apparently because moderate drinkers generally enjoy socializing, engage in life-enhancing interests, and derive the health benefits of alcohol.

Studies consistently show that moderate drinkers have less heart disease. Many drinkers stop drinking because they have medical complications, and heavy drinkers are at a high risk of organic disturbance and disease. But social drinkers, who make up the vast majority, should be glad to know that moderate drinking is not only good for them but does no harm.

Most abstainers do not drink for moral, ethical, or health reasons. Other abstainers are "social dropouts," who withdraw from established society. The decision to eschew social and emotional contact may partly explain the difference between the life spans of abstainers and moderate drinkers.

Despite these statistics, people cannot be generalized, and hundreds of individual responses pop up to defy the statisticians. The solace and support that abstainers find in following their religious or ethical principles are more important to their well-being than the statistical probability of longer life with moderate drinking.

So far the findings are very comforting to the moderate drinker.

How does alcohol affect the heart?

It is universally known today that moderate drinkers have less heart disease than heavy drinkers or abstainers. Moreover, people who have heart disease benefit from moderate amounts of alcohol. Many heart patients find that a little alcohol relieves the painful grip of angina. The vasodilation property of alcohol permits the blood to flow more freely.

Alcohol's analgesic qualities quiet the natural anxiety of the heart patient who wonders if every twinge of pain in the chest heralds disaster. Moreover, sudden cardiac arrest is rarer among moderate drinkers than abstainers. The relaxation effect of mild amounts of alcohol may speed the recovery of the cardiac patient.

How does alcohol affect the brain?

All of your incoming sensations travel along nerve fibers in the brain. The cerebral cortex is the conscious and thinking overseer of the brain, while other sites control automatic activities. The nervous system is often described as a chain of switching devices with junctions along the way to direct the traffic of incoming stimuli. Incoming stimuli must overcome resistance at the junctions that are called "threshold resistances." The resistance slows down the energy of the incoming stimulus. At this point in the journey, it is theorized, the action of alcohol affects the incoming sensations in one of two ways: it slows down their rate of speed or, with heavy amounts, prevents the sensations from entering the brain entirely.

Is alcohol good for the elderly?

The elderly population is the fastest-growing segment of the nation's population. As your longevity increases, your exposure to health risks increases, and everyday problems such as disturbed digestion, joint and muscle pains, feelings of isolation and uselessness, and the need for medication become lifestyle eroders. Because of its mild anesthetic effect, occasional small amounts of alcohol can lessen the drain of everyday aches and pains.

Is alcohol medication?

Alcohol is a basic ingredient in the preparation of liquid medications and tonics. Historically, it has been used alone as a medicine. Before antibiotics, physicians prescribed small amounts of whiskey for infants suffering from pneumonia. And cowboy heroes could not have withstood the pain of a bullet extraction without heavy gulps of alcohol.

Today, alcohol is used on chronic disease wards in hospitals to ease patient discomfort and to give them something to think about besides their illness.

Many tonics advertised and sold over-the-counter as medication to help your blood or relieve infirmities owe their success in part to alcohol in the mixture.

Does alcohol improve the appetite?

Alcohol stimulates the appetite by affecting the brain's inhibitory centers. When sensations of fatigue, jaded taste, and nervous indigestion suppress the appetite, the effects of alcohol can make the food begin to smell, look, and taste better. Certainly, alcohol weakens the will to resist eating.

Does alcohol aid digestion?

Historically, small amounts of alcohol were taken before meals to aid digestion. Beer and wine are particularly useful for this purpose because of their compatibility with the stomach's gastric juices.

The acid content of wine, for example, is close to the acid content of the stomach. Alcohol's mild anesthetic effect improves the "dry mouth" syndrome associated with stress or tension, and your mouth begins to salivate more freely. Salivation, in turn, triggers motility—the gentle motion that empties the stomach and is considered beneficial to digestion. One or two glasses of wine with a meal can produce this effect.

Heavy amounts are another story and cause both an irritated stomach wall and an increased concentration of alcohol. An anesthetized stomach is too sleepy to move or is so overwrought it tightens up in a spasm.

Is it okay to drink a little when I have an ulcer?

You should not drink alcohol if you have an ulcer. The raw, exposed stomach tissue does not take kindly to alcohol's acidic content. In fact, it's foolish and dangerous to drink while you have an ulcer.

Will alcohol help me sleep?

A small amount of alcohol taken about a half-hour before retiring can relieve tension and induce sleep. It is not recommended as a daily practice, because should you need to increase the amount, the opposite will occur: uneven, poor sleep. With heavy amounts of alcohol, you will sleep fitfully and wake up exhausted. This sleep disturbance is caused by a decrease of REM (rapid eye movement) or dreaming sleep. You need a certain amount of REM sleep each night. Without it, you'll have difficulty with your concentration and memory, and you'll feel anxious, tired, and irritable. Alcohol in large amounts blocks REM sleep as it narcotizes the control centers that regulate sleep and dreaming.

Probably the best way to induce sleep is not to focus on it. Read, work, and don't fight it. People fuss about getting enough sleep, but I've never heard of an insomniac dying for lack of it, and many people function perfectly well with only a few hours of sleep a night.

How does drinking affect nutrition?

Alcohol affects your nutrition only a little when you drink within Anstie's limits. You may have a bit more fat floating around in your blood and even being deposited temporarily in your liver. Although the reason for floating fat is not totally understood, it's attributed to the process of alcohol oxidation that releases an excess of hydrogen in the liver. The increase in hydrogen is thought to inhibit certain metabolic functions helpful in deriving energy from other sources, making alcohol the "preferred fuel" for energy. The hydrogen also frees fat from other parts of the body to float in the blood. Although this fat settles temporarily in the liver, it disappears within twenty-four hours after drinking. For some reason not understood, not all the unused calories provided by alcohol get stored as fat, as do nutritional calories.

Heavy drinking is another matter. Your taste buds are so anesthetized that either you don't eat or you don't eat properly. Heavy drinking upsets the body's metabolism and disturbs the absorption processes of your digestive system. You are unable to extract all the necessary nutrients from the food you have consumed. Heavy amounts of alcohol are bad enough, but when heavy drinking causes nutritional deficiencies, the worst complications of alcoholism begin.

Some researchers contend that only the nutritional deficits lead to ill health, not the alcohol. This is a foolish differentiation. Even if you eat properly but drink heavily, you so upset complicated metabolic mechanisms that nutritional pandemonium breaks out.

Does a drinking spree present any special health hazards?

Whenever you become intoxicated, you are flirting with danger. If the truth be known, a strong possibility exists that you will have an experience sometime with overdrinking. A drinking spree can constitute a personal and social threat. If and when this happens make sure you are in a protected environment.

Because you have overdosed with alcohol, the civilized part of the brain is affected by the anesthetic property of alcohol, and the primitive part of the brain takes over. When this toxic phenomenon happens, you are out of control.

What are the adverse physical effects of heavy drinking?

Heavy drinking adversely affects the brain, nerves, muscles, stomach, and throat. We do not know if the harm is done by nutritional deficiencies or by the heavy intake of alcohol directly. I believe that most researchers still buy nutritional interference rather than direct alcohol action. One thing everyone agrees on is that heavy drinking is not good for your health.

Most investigators are not convinced that cirrhosis of the liver is caused directly by heavy doses of alcohol. In an interesting study by a New York group, thirteen baboons were fed large quantities of alcohol along with adequate diets. Two cirrhotic livers resulted. Unfortunately, the study did not measure whether the baboons' heavy alcoholic intake interfered with their ability to absorb the nutritious diet.

The New York group claims that its study proves direct effects because it controlled the experiment with a properly balanced diet. Whether these claims are correct, there is no doubt that heavy drinkers put their livers at risk, and the consensus is if you drink heavily, you are better off if you eat an adequate nutritious diet.

Chapter 9

Alcohol and Your Feelings

Throughout history and around the world, alcohol has been used to alter reality, quiet fears, and soothe anxieties.

Why does alcohol make me feel more relaxed and uninhibited?

Alcohol makes you feel more relaxed and uninhibited because the new part of the brain that controls tension and inhibitions is sensitive to alcohol.

When you drink alcohol, the activity of the newer brain center slows down. Social controls relax. You're less tense, less inhibited, freer. In a sense, you are a trifle less civilized and a trifle more yourself. That's amore!

Why do I get *more* depressed if I drink?

I'd advise you to stop drinking if you get more depressed when you drink. Drinking is for reaching out, not for reaching in. If your depression intensifies with alcohol, your depression is serious, and you need professional help.

When alcohol increases depression, drinkers tend to take more to medicate the depression. The problem here is lack of experience and knowledge. Depression can be successfully treated.

During chaotic times, is there an increase in the national consumption of alcohol?

Some studies show that during periods of national crises, people buy more alcohol. For example, in a depressed economy, consumption rates tend to rise.

Why do I occasionally feel that I *need* a drink?

Some time or other you may reach a point of exhaustion or tension that leads you to seek the relaxing properties of alcohol. Feeling the need for a drink is an expression of the human experience.

If the world and its people were perfect, you would never *need* anything. However, claiming to need a drink puts alcohol into a functional role that is potentially dangerous. If you frequently say, "Boy, do I *need* a drink," it's an expression of a need to be dependent. It's time to be cautious. Become dependent on something other than alcohol.

When you drink only for the anesthetic effect, you will gradually require increasing amounts to achieve the original response. That's how dependency problems with alcohol begin.

Why can I feel close to certain people only when I drink?

Some people have been raised to repress feelings of warmth and closeness. These patterns of restraint become a part of their nature. Even when they intellectually want to feel close, they can't.

A moderate amount of alcohol releases uptight social controls and makes expressing the innate human impulse to be close to people quite natural.

Chapter 10

Alcohol and Drugs

Mixing alcohol and drugs can have unexpected, often devastating and sometimes lethal effects. An important rule of thumb for sensible social drinking is to know which medications can be safely taken with alcohol and which cannot.

Is mixing alcohol and drugs really that dangerous?

Mixing alcohol and drugs can have many undesirable effects. Alcohol can diminish a drug's effectiveness, increase its toxicity, or be a relatively harmless companion. Where there is an interaction, the combination can produce one of two outcomes. The first is called an *additive response*. This means a half dose of each drug produces the cumulative effect of a full dose of each. The second is called a *potentiating response*. This means a synergistic action is produced when two drugs are combined resulting in a greater effect than a full dose of either drug.

Even small amounts of alcohol combined with

drugs can send you to the hospital. If you're taking medication, I recommend you ask your doctor or pharmacist about how it will affect you if you drink.

Are some drugs more dangerous with alcohol than others?

Physicians commonly warn against the use of alcohol with barbiturates, such as the phenobarbitals, sedatives such as Dalmane, and antihistamines such as Benadryl. The dangers of combining alcohol with *some* medication can be serious and very risky. For instance, taking a popular tranquilizer or an over-the-counter antihistamine can compromise your acuity and contribute to poor driving performance.

Even familiar analgesic drugs like the salicylates such as aspirin, with continuous use, tend to produce bleeding in the stomach, and irritation from alcohol would aggravate the condition. Heavy amounts of alcohol taken with salicylates can overwhelm the body's blood-clotting mechanism and cause hemorrhaging.

On the other hand, Tylenol (acetaminophen) does not bother the stomach. It is reported that heavy alcohol use and lots of Tylenol may cause liver damage.

Probably the best rule to follow is not to drink alcohol while taking any medication; but since only a few stalwarts exercise such discipline, you should make it your business to know the risks of mixing alcohol with medications.

What are the effects of specific medications when combined with alcohol?[1]

Some concurrent use of alcohol and medicinal drugs is inevitable. The following drugs are but a sampling of the vast pharmacopeia of available medications.

The ubiquitous **Antibiotic** is an example of frequent concurrent use with alcohol. Known as the "wonder drug" of earlier decades, antibiotics are used to fight infections caused by bacteria. Such drugs include the penicillins, sulfonamides, tetracyclines, and miscellaneous antibiotics such as chloromycetin. Taken with antibiotics, alcohol has no significant interaction for most people. In very rare cases, concurrent use causes flushing, headache, nausea, and vomiting.

Anticoagulants such as heparin and warfarin are drugs used to prevent clots from forming or from spreading. They are commonly prescribed for people who suffer a heart attack or a stroke due to blocked vessels. There are no significant interactions between alcohol and anticoagulants.

---

[1] A major resource for the information in this section was a paper entitled "Medical Consequences of Alcohol-Drug Interactions" by Brian F. Sands, M.D., Clifford M. Knapp, Ph.D., and Domenic A. Ciraulo, M.D., which appeared in the Spring 1994 edition of *Alcohol Health and Research World.*

Medicines called **Anticonvulsants** such as Dilantin, benzodiazepines, barbiturates, and others are used to treat people with seizure disorders. Alcohol may cause an increase in the elimination of anticonvulsants from the body, thereby increasing the risk of seizures.

Nonsteroidal   Anti-Inflammatory   Drugs (NSAIDs) are medications used to treat inflammation, pain, and fever. Aspirin, Motrin, ibuprofen, and the like can increase stomach irritation, and with alcohol use can lead to severe stomach pain and even gastric bleeding.

Antidepressants are used to treat depressive disorders. Alcohol has a significant interaction with antidepressants of the tricyclic class such as amitriptyline (Elavil and others) and doxepin (Sinequan and others) causing increased impairment of muscular movement. The highly publicized antidepressant Prozac (fluoxetine) does not appear to have much of an interaction with alcohol.

Aromatic chemicals found in some beer and wine (but not alcohol itself) can elevate blood pressure in people taking monoamine oxidase inhibitors: tranylcypromine (Parnate), phenelzine (Nardil), and isocarboxazid (Marplan).

When taking **Sedatives and Hypnotics** (sleeping pills) with alcohol, real care must be exercised. For example, the benzodiazepines that treat anxiety and insomnia are also used as anticonvulsants and as adjuncts to anesthesia. The benzodiazepines include diazepam (Valium), chlordiazepoxide (Librium), alprazolam (Xanax) loraxepam (Ativan), and temazepam (Restoril). The interaction between alcohol and benzodiazapines may be additive or synergistic and can lead to diminished alertness and function. The inability to function properly can occur with just standard doses of benzodiazepines and small amounts of alcohol.

In the past few years, barbiturates have taken a backseat to the benzodiazepines. Barbiturates are now used less for sleep induction and more for the prevention and emergency treatment of seizures. Some common barbiturates are butalbital (Fiorinal and others), meprobamate (Miltown and others) pentobarbital (Nemutal), phenobarbital (Donnatal and others), and secobarbital (Seconal). Barbiturates interact with alcohol to cause additive or synergistic decreases in alertness and motor skills.

Calcium Channel Blockers such as verapamil (Calan and others), diltiazem (Cardizem and others), and nifedipine (Procardia and others) are prescribed for people with high blood pressure, abnormal heart beat, or angina. These drugs are used to block the passage of calcium into the muscle cells of the heart and blood vessels. There is no known interaction between these drugs and alcohol in humans.

Cocaine and marijuana (cannabis) have an additive action with alcohol causing a diminished ability to function. We do not know the mechanism for this interaction.

Alcohol can increase the cocaine "high." It interacts synergistically to increase the heart rate and may increase cocaine's toxic effects on the liver.

Antihistamines such as cimetidine (Tagamet) and ranitidine (Zantac) reduce the acid secretions of the stomach and thus increase the potential of alcohol. Other histamine antagonists such as diphenhydramine (Benadryl and others) can cause increased sedative action when combined with alcohol. They are used to allieviate symptoms of the common cold, allergies, and the like.

Antipsychotics are medications used to treat serious mental illnesses such as schizophrenia and manic depression. Acute alcohol consumption with the antipsychotic drug chlorpromazine can decrease the elimination of chlorpromazine (Thorazine) leading to higher levels of the drug in the body and attendant risks of serious side effects.

Opioids are drugs used for pain relief. Combined with alcohol, drugs such as propoxyphene (Darvon, morphine, and others) increase the risk of severe sedation, coma, and respiratory arrest.

Antidiabetics such as insulin, taken by mouth or by injection, combined with alcohol can lead to severe hypoglycemia, in other words, an exaggerated insulin response.

An **Antialcoholic** drug used to enforce abstinence is called Antabuse (disulfiram). When Antabuse is combined with alcohol it produces a very unpleasant feeling of flushing, painful throbbing in the head and neck, headaches, difficulty in breathing, nausea and vomiting, and almost any other uncomfortable symptom you can imagine.

Diuretics such as thiazide (Diuril and others) or quinethazone (Hydromox) appear to have no problem with the concurrent use of alcohol. Some people contend that retaining water may be one of the major problems of chronic heavy drinkers, and since diuretics help eliminate water, diuretics may even be helpful.

Chapter 11

You and Alcohol and People

Alcohol is an excellent catalyst for social interaction. Whether you use it or abuse it will depend on your attitude, on the attitude of the company you keep, and most of all on the attitude of the society in which you live.

The company you keep

Most people behave in an acceptable fashion not because of rules, regulations, and laws, but because they need the affection and respect of a few individuals around them. These individuals consciously and unconsciously transmit the limits of behavior they will expect and accept from you. You make sure not to tamper with these limits, if you want to continue the relationships.

Therefore, in a given situation where an individual in your group is misusing alcohol, what should you do? First, you should understand that your friend is dealing with a serious problem. And second, ask yourself what role you play in influencing your friend to solve a problem by abusing alcohol.

Drinking together

Thousands of years ago, when your ancestors found the world even more mystifying than you do today, men and women lived in terror of the forces that seemed to control their fate. The use of alcohol made it possible not only to tolerate these forces but also to gain a sense of mastery over them. In this way alcohol took its place in social and religious ritual.

Pagan religion, like modern religion, was part social, part mystical. Members gathered for mutual support. Soon after alcohol became acculturated, it was used to ratify contracts, solemnize crownings, mark festive events, and confirm all rites of passage through life. Today alcohol is used to celebrate the birth of a child, entry into college, hopes for a happy marriage, a new job, and new partnerships. Even death and mourning are softened by drinking.

Wine enhances food's natural flavor, heightens its aroma, and increases one's gustatory pleasure. The Bible mentions alcohol's appeal to the appetite: "Drink no longer water, but use a little wine for thy stomach's sake."

Expressions of hospitality, sociability, and conviviality would be incomplete in some circles without alcohol. Alcohol in small amounts allows the shy person to speak, the sexually constricted to respond, and can reaffirm affection and real friendship.

Group drinking has a broader significance than the mere consumption of alcohol at an event, party, or sporting venue. For example, pubs in England are really social clubs for meeting and entertaining friends and acquantances. They are living rooms for lonely people. An expression of such a phenomenon is even seen on Skid Row. Although Skid Row drinking groups usually gather at mutual watering holes, just the act of assembling becomes a bond of cohesiveness for these social outcasts.

When you drink to get in touch with other people, you are drinking for the best reason.

Why am I friendlier when I drink?

When you drink you're less self-conscious, less serious, less self-impressed. In moderate doses, alcohol becomes a leveler, a socializer. When alcohol gently relaxes the stern forms of "new" brain control, the dormant humanistic impulses are expressed as friendliness.

At some parties everyone has a good time, and no one gets drunk; at other parties the same people get drunk and act like fools. Why?

Each party is set up for its outcome. At some parties you, the host, transmit the message clearly. By serving no food, you're saying alcohol is all. By topping off drinks as they dip below the rim, you're saying alcohol is all. By pushing people to drink when they're not in the mood, you're telling them to get drunk.

At other parties, cocktails and hors d'oeuvres are offered for a limited time, and guests are not urged to drink. Dinner is served on time, and seating is arranged for conversation. The noise level is low and the lights are soft. The focus is on people, not alcohol. Alcohol is the accompaniment, not the preoccupation. The host's message is: Have a good time, but don't get drunk.

The basic influence at work here in both instances is expectation. When you drink, you ordinarily get the response you, or those around you, expect.

Why do I feel more comfortable at a party where others are making fools of themselves?

Some people are tragically self-conscious. They are, as one patient confessed, corseted by the belief that the lights and cameras are focused on them alone. Actually, they dread center stage. If someone acts the fool at a party, they feel more comfortable, because the possibility of their being noticed has shifted to the fool.

Why is it so hard not to drink at a cocktail party?

It's not unlike being at a movie and not looking. A party named after a drink implies a celebration of alcohol. If you don't drink, you feel left out, especially if the host and guests eye you as being unsociable. It is a trying situation. The trick, of course, is to have *something* in your glass to sip on, e.g., a Virgin Mary, club soda and orange juice, Perrier and lime, 7-Up and grenadine, iced tea, lemonade, tonic and lime, or a Virgin Colada.

Does peer pressure make people drink?

You are influenced by certain people in your life whose respect, affection, and acceptance you desire and need. I call it peer need, not peer pressure.

These people set limits (formally or informally) on how far you can go and what they'll tolerate. If the relationship is good, they cannot force you to do something you don't want to do. They share your view of the world, your cares, your pleasures, and they provide support, comfort, and a reality check.

To be pressured to drink or to act against your better judgment is neither caring nor sharing—it is using. Unfortunately, our peer needs sometimes make it very hard to resist destructive pressures.

What is the relationship between religious affiliation and drinking?

Religious affiliation often offers some protection against an alcohol problem. The wholehearted acceptance of religious dogma by members of a religious group is a combination of personal conviction and peer need. In denominations whose strictures against alcohol are especially strong, most of the members do not drink. But when they do, they are likely to develop problems with alcohol.

Chapter 12

Your Drinking Heritage

Drinking behavior reflects national, ethnic, and philosophical approaches to drinking.

How does the American value system affect my drinking habits?

The United States is a country that revels in abundance. Its people produce and drive a monumental number of cars. Its food supply and resource production are bountiful. The American home showcases the latest high-tech products in every room. Americans consume prodigiously, and when they eat and drink, their behavior reflects the emphasis on bountiful consumption.

What do the problem-drinking nations have in common?

I don't know which among the problem-drinking nations (United States, France, Sweden, and Russia) is "better" and which is "worse." As best we know, Russia, which has a historical problem with alcohol abuse, has today serious social problems with alcohol resulting from the breakup of the Soviet empire. In my opinion, Russia has the most serious alcohol problems of the developed world.

The United States, Sweden, and Russia suffer from the same problems with alcohol use, and for similar reasons—their people do not know how to drink. They drink fast and impatiently; they use drinking to prove their prowess; they focus on alcohol; they ascribe undeserved magical qualities to it; they often drink without food; and drunkenness is implicitly and explicitly approved. It's also important to note that the United States, Sweden, and Russia have high rates of depression.

France's problem is somewhat different. French people, particularly the working class, honestly believe that water is unsafe and that wine is good for the blood. They use wine to quench thirst as well as to accompany meals, and sip, at intervals, all day long. For many Frenchmen, the day routinely begins with cognac and coffee. Though the roaring drunk is rare, the quiet drunk is common, and alcohol problems are widespread.

What about American drinking patterns?

The per capita consumption rate of alcohol is known only by published tax figures on sales of alcohol. According to these figures, Washington, D.C. has a higher per capita consumption rate than that of all other measured locales, and this estimate does not include the tax-free purchases of foreign embassies. Does this mean we have a capital city of heavy drinkers? Not at all. These figures can be misleading.

Washington has no rural area to dilute its population. Moreover, it is a convention and tourist center, and people tend to drink more and more often while at conventions and on vacation. Moreover, Washington is a relatively low-cost liquor spot, so bargain hunters come to the District from surrounding Virginia and Maryland to buy alcohol. The high figures don't necessarily indicate that Washington residents are heavy drinkers.

American drinking tastes have shifted over the years. One hundred and fifty years ago, distilled spirits accounted for 90 percent of the alcohol consumed in this country. Now it is less than half of that, with beer sales taking up most of the slack. Beer now is the most popular alcoholic beverage in America.

Americans are drinking less today than they did in 1981 but more than they did in 1950. This is mostly attributable to two major population trends: the baby-boomer bonanza after World War II, and the rapidly increasing elderly population.

However, worldwide sales of alcohol today are flat or falling.

What effect did the American occupation of Japan after World War II have on Japanese drinking habits?

The Japanese experience strongly indicates that alcohol problems are learned, not inherited. Before World

War II, the Japanese were models of responsible drinking behavior. While drinking was common, drunkenness and drinking problems were not.

During the American occupation, the Japanese people adopted many American customs, including our way of drinking. The civilized milieu of the geisha house was replaced by American-style cocktail bars and the ubiquitous hostesses. Drunkenness was common, and alcohol problems became a concern to the Japanese people. Getting drunk after work became a daily ritual for many Japanese white-collar workers.

Why do Native Americans and the Irish have a notoriously high rate of alcoholism?

The common denominator is deprivation. The Native Americans were deprived of their culture, their land, their pride, their physical well-being, their dignity. They were also deprived of the opportunity to learn how to drink. Giving alcohol to an unpracticed, physically and emotionally deprived people is like giving candy to a baby.

The Irish did have practice in drinking, but for the wrong reasons and in the wrong way. The Irish were deprived of heterosexual exposure and economic opportunity. Irish mothers approved of their boys' getting drunk at the bar—it meant they weren't getting in trouble with women. Irish fathers also sanctioned their boys' getting drunk. In rural Ireland, the farm was the family's only economic resource, and it didn't necessarily go to the oldest son upon the death of the father. The father usually kept the choice to himself as long as possible to keep all his sons at home. Drunken sprees helped the boys bear the uncertainty.

Why do the French, but not the Italians, have serious alcohol problems, when both give their children alcohol at an early age?

Alcohol is introduced to an Italian child as just another part of eating and socializing. Italian parents take food, sip a little wine, talk and laugh a little, but they don't get drunk.

French children learn that wine is the beverage of choice, because water is unsafe and milk is indigestible to anyone beyond the age of six months. Moreover, French children see around them people who drink continuously. They grow up with this image of drinking behavior.

As you will note in the next question, ethnicity can be protective; assimilation into a larger culture dilutes that protection. With global communication so widespread, ethnic values disappear into a "world" culture. Fortunately or unfortunately, the American way has become the role model for drinking behavior among developed nations. As a consequence, French children are more attracted to soft drinks than to wine.

What ethnic groups in America are least likely to become alcoholic?

First-generation Italians, Jews, and Chinese are unlikely to become alcoholic. As a matter of fact, if the Italian remains within an Italian setting, and the Jew clings to his orthodoxy, and the Chinese resist assimilation, alcoholism is extremely rare among them.

However, as the second generation becomes Americanized, it more often takes on American drinking behavior and abandons its ethnic drinking culture. Still, second-generation Chinese, Italians, and Jews do not feel kindly toward drunkenness. For them, moderate consumption of alcohol is the norm.

By the third generation, however, the dilution of ethnic values is greater. A night on the town once in a while is not uncommon. Socialization with the focus on heavy drinking is tolerated. American drinking habits have replaced ethnic values. Alcoholic people with Jewish, Italian, and Chinese names are beginning to show up at AA meetings.

Chapter 13

On the Job

In many ways your work defines you. Your social status, your friends, even your family relations depend on the work you do. Add to this the traditions, expectations, and pressures of the work-a-day world, and it's easy to see that your job can influence the way you drink.

Alcohol in business—good or bad?

Alcohol is standard equipment in business and professional life. For example, where I live in Washington, D.C., socializing is an extension of office hours—only the venue changes. Away from the office, information is exchanged, pacts are made, business relations are formed. Alcohol becomes a useful catalyst, and the social setting condones its use.

As a result, drinking is an accompaniment to business functions. Certainly the Washington scene is not unique, but wherever it exists, be wary of the crutch.

Alcohol is a useful adjunct to business in social

functions. However, when it is used in order to function better professionally—watch out. For instance, if you use alcohol regularly to keep your tension level in control, or drink before difficult meetings to bolster your confidence or to relieve early morning nerves, you ought to check your reality level. It may indicate a disability. You may be using alcohol as a crutch to perform.

Do the military services have unusual drinking problems?

Studies indicate a serious misuse of alcohol and a large number of alcohol problems in the military. People in the services drink because alcohol is offered as part of the accepted array of opportunities to exhibit maturity and strength. The attitudes that condone heavy alcohol use need to be reexamined for both the well-being of the troops and the military's effectiveness.

In what other fields do you see alcoholic people?

According to the American Medical Association, the practice of medicine loses four hundred doctors each year to alcoholism. What's more, these highly esteemed members of the community need to be obviously sick before anyone will help, notice, or diagnose them. That's a lot of wasted talent—almost three full medical-school graduating classes.

In the nineteenth century, the only major American writer known to suffer from a severe alcohol problem was Edgar Allan Poe. In the twentieth century, the number of writers known to have severe alcohol problems is staggering.

In the world of sports, people make inordinate demands on their heroes. The pressure to perform drives many performers to seek the anesthetic solace of alcohol.

Why do so many people in powerful positions have drinking problems?

Power, itself, is an intoxicant. People who wield power tend to operate in the worlds of influence and super-human feats.

Powerful people are courted at parties and lionized in public. Many of them use alcohol to deal with the mental and physical tensions of power.

A member of Congress once said publicly, "There is no better training ground for alcoholism than serving in the Congress of the United States." Heavy drinking is an occupational hazard inherent to all power centers.

Why do spouses of famous people have drinking problems?

Fame exacts a price. Famous people and their families must constantly live up to an image fantasized by their adoring fans. The reward is adulation and recognition. The penalty is a false front.

The spouse, as a mere appendage, suffers an even greater loss of identity than the famed mate, and any satisfactions are, at best, vicarious. Vicarious pleasures are poor food for the human spirit. The hunger to be recognized as an individual is sated by heavy amounts of alcohol. In pursuing that occupation, one identity is easy to achieve—that of an alcoholic.

Why do many homemakers have a drinking problem?

Boredom and feelings of uselessness are the enemies of sanity. Whenever personal terrors prey on people, they divert their aloneness and anxiety by seeking useful occupations that make them feel wanted and needed.

Homemakers who are not able to escape confinement begin to depend on frequent amounts of alcohol. In the reveries of heavy drinking, boredom and despondency melt away, temporarily.

Why do certain kinds of work have a higher rate of alcoholism?

The demands of the job and a ready exposure to alcohol can increase your risk of alcoholism. Studies show that the setting and circumstance are often more at fault for developing alcohol problems than are individual psychological needs.

Certain professions such as the theater, television, professional sports, politics, magazine and newspaper work—jobs with tight deadlines, public exposure, and the pressure to excel are high tension producers. Some people use alcohol to socialize, to entertain clients and colleagues, to social climb, to woo important people. Also, some jobs are just boring and lonely, and the people engaged in them use alcohol to relieve the daily drudge.

No one knows whether the profession facilitates the onset and course of an individual's alcohol problem or whether the individual chooses the profession that makes it easy to develop alcohol problems.

What are the business advantages, if any, to drinking?

In our society, there are individuals who view non-drinkers as people struggling with an alcohol problem or as finger-pointing teetotallers. They consider abstainers unfriendly, afraid to let down their hair, and secretive. Perhaps the business advantage to drinking in this instance might be to avoid suspicious looks. Today, however, it is perfectly acceptable and respectable to say that you are a recovering alcoholic or that you simply choose not to drink.

Chapter 14

Your Children

National attitudes, peer group standards, and family values will shape your children's drinking patterns, just as they shaped yours.

If my teenager drinks, is he or she an alcoholic?

People assume that occasional bouts of excessive drinking during adolescence will inevitably lead to alcoholism. They logically make this assumption when the household composition shows an alcoholic parent or other problem drinkers in the family. Moreover, studies continue to link the drinking practices of teenagers with the abusive behavior of the problem drinker. Most parents, who stand in awe and in fear of their offspring anyway, think that drinking during the "terrible teens" will certainly lead to drunkenness and alcoholism.

Now let us separate fact from myth. *Teenage drinking is not alcoholism.* Teenage drinking is the experimental use of alcohol by boys and girls in their teens, not the abusive drinking of an alcoholic. I am not talking here about unhealthy social, physical, or economic adjustment to alcohol. So it's important that you make a distinction between alcoholism and teenage drinking—the former is a serious medical problem. Teenage drinking is not.

An effective method that advocacy groups use to create an antialcohol climate is to frighten the public about the behavior of their children. The teenage years are frightening for the parents, the children, and society. And the thought that your teenager is engaging in the same risky behavior that you did when you were a teenager—especially with alcohol and sex—is hard to take. Fortunately, and despite the doomspreaders, you survived the terrible teens; so will your kids.

Is my concern about teenage behavior a new problem?

The concern you have about your children is not new. According to the inscription on an Assyrian tablet in 2800 B.C., an ancient lamented: "Our earth is degenerate in these latter days. Bribery and corruption are common. Children no longer obey their parents."

A few centuries later, Socrates further commented that children pursued luxury, showed disrespect for their parents, and tyrannized their elders. Times haven't changed.

Adolescence is a complex and confusing time, and parents figuratively cross their fingers. Statistics show teens more at risk for suicide than any other segment of the population. But don't be too hard on yourself. A teenager vascillates between being a child and a grown-up.

Adolescence is a period of transition, insecurity, and strain for both adolescents and those around them. The uncertainty of the age is caused, on the one hand, by the natural urge to become independent of family while learning about responsibility. On the other hand, teenagers still want the comforts of a protective environment.

Sociologists label the sudden and abrupt press for independence a rite of passage in our society. Other societies have formal, ceremonial rites of passage to celebrate the transition from child to adult.

Should I teach my children to drink? What should I tell them?

If you drink, you *are* teaching your children to drink. All studies confirm that parents are the most important role models for their children. The way you drink is likely to be the way they will drink. A drinking parent will likely have a drinking offspring.

Children learn about alcohol very early in life.

They notice the way their parents and friends act when they drink alcohol—they notice that it's treated as something special. Most parents respond to children who ask to taste something they eat or drink. But when children ask to taste alcohol, without recognizing the inconsistency, parents say, "You can't have it because it's not good for you." *This is education.*

Your children learn about alcohol from the outside world. A party dress is called a cocktail dress. Some events are named after alcohol—cocktail parties, beer busts, wine-tasting parties, and so forth. Songs are related to alcohol. Magazines, television, and sporting events are resplendent with advertisements for alcohol. Children incorporate these signals. *This is education.*

Parents can do little about signals from the world at large, but at home you have the best opportunity to teach them by natural example. For instance, when you're drinking, give them a sip if they ask to taste it, but caution them that they may not like the taste.

Other cultures give alcohol to their young in the family setting without a fuss and without appreciable problems. Common sense and your own intuition is still the best formula. Remove the mystery, defuse the allure, break down the barriers, and set limits appropriate to age and development. Do you know anyone who struggles very hard for what he or she can easily get?

When children ask about alcohol, give them the facts included in this book. But telling is less important than showing. The best education is to set an example by the way you drink.

Do the children of alcoholic parents have a higher rate of alcoholism than the children of nonalcoholic parents?

Children of alcoholic parents are more likely to develop alcohol problems than children of nonalcoholic parents. The alcohol problems of adult children of alcoholics can be considered as *learned* behavior.

Society, in coming to grips with the safe use of alcohol as well as its problems, must deal with the "contagion" factor. We think contagious refers only to disease spread through germs. But learned, unhealthy, dangerous behavior is just as contagious, just as sickness-producing.

If parents can spread dysfunctional and debilitating ways of living, doesn't it follow that they can transmit healthy, responsible ones as well? As people learn how to use alcohol as it should be used, their children will have good examples to follow.

Can teenagers really handle alcohol?

I know of nothing about alcohol or teenagers that would preclude their handling alcohol well. In drinking, as in most things, experience, responsibility, and self-respect tend to lead to a favorable outcome. Young people haven't had the time or opportunity to gain much experience, so be sure you provide favorable circumstances, preferably at home, for them to practice their drinking.

When teenagers begin to drink, why do they booze it up?

Young people look at drinking as a major rite of passage from childhood to adulthood. Unfortunately society has made alcohol forbidden and special by raising the drinking age to 21.

Proponents of "21" point to a reduction in the incidence of teenage accident rates as proof that raising the drinking age works. However, Canada had a similiar drop in accidents among teenagers, and the drinking age throughout the Canadian provinces is 18 or 19. As unpracticed, sereptitious drinkers, teenagers believe having a good time with alcohol means getting drunk. Young people equate boozed up with grown up. No one shows them the safe way to drink.

In some groups, boozed up means belonging. At that uncertain age, to them belonging—even to the point of having to get drunk—is worth the misery and risk of overdrinking.

Do the youth of other countries have drinking problems?

Some do. The drunkenness of Russian youth is called hooliganism. Swedish young people get drunk often, too. If a country's adult population has drinking problems, it's a sure bet that a like proportion of its young people do, too.

Chapter 15

Drinking and Driving

If you pay attention to your response to alcohol, you will know from the first sip to the last drop whether your response is normal and safe.

How many drinks can I have and still drive safely?

In the American style of oversimplification, the issue of *drunk* driving became an issue of *drinking* and driving. Drinking and driving is *not* the same as drunk driving.

The important point to remember when drinking is your response to alcohol, not the amount of alcohol. If you pay attention to your response to alcohol when you drink, you'll know from the first sip to the last drop whether your response is normal and safe for you.

Since alcohol can occasionally fool even the experienced drinker, people are being trained in the TIPS program (noted below) to prevent you from doing harm to yourself or others.

111

What is BAC?

BAC (blood-alcohol concentration) refers to your blood-alcohol level. For legal purposes, most states consider a level of 0.1 BAC as *legal* intoxication (some states have already lowered it to 0.08). If Anstie's limit is observed with slow drinking, the BAC should not reach a level beyond 0.05. Many studies on BAC readings and driving do not differentiate between the incidence of accidents at the 0.05 level and the incidence of accidents of the nondrinker.

How much does it really take to impair my driving ability?

An average-size person who *quickly* swallows three shots of whiskey, or five cans of beer, or four glasses of wine is impaired for driving. Any drinking that pushes your blood-alcohol level (BAC) above 0.05 begins to affect driving skills. The higher the blood-alcohol level, the greater the risk. By the time your BAC reaches 0.1, you're *legally* intoxicated.

Are the Breathalyzer and urine tests unfair?

The Breathalyzer, even with its imperfections (a strong odor of garlic, emphysema, and bronchitis can cause a false reading), is generally a reliable approach for identifying drunk drivers. What's more, its popular use shows you that society disapproves of individuals who drive while drunk. People believe that drinking is a matter of choice, but driving is a privilege that does not include the right to endanger others.

I think urine tests are unfair, because they don't accurately measure the level of alcohol.

How many accidents in the United States are related to alcohol?

Heavy drinking and accidents show a high correlation in the United States. Twenty-two percent of all traffic fatalities on the highway are caused by heavy alcohol users. However, the statistics become skewed when a person with even a smidgen of alcohol in the blood, such as 0.01 BAC, has an accident and it is labeled as alcohol-related. Antialcohol advocates falsely use any "alcohol-related" statistic as evidence to condemn alcohol as the cause of accidents. To be truly fair, statistics should also record accidents as weather-related, fatigue-related, stress-related, food-related, etc.

What can I do about drunk driving?

Only a fool would allow an acquaintance who is drunk to drive a car. Sensible, experienced drinkers know when to stop drinking if they are driving. Likewise, they can recognize when someone else is unfit to drive.

The first thing you can do to help is accept the fact that people sometimes drink too much. The second thing involves action. If someone you know is unfit to drive, call a cab, offer a ride home, take away the keys, do anything to prevent the possibility of an accident.

What can bars do about drunk driving?

A likely place to abuse alcohol is at the ubiquitous bar. People go to bars for diversion: to drink, to eat, and to talk; then, they drive home. The slogan "Friends don't let friends drive drunk" is good advice and a useful sound bite, but it doesn't tell you what to do and how to do it.

Out in the work-a-day world, a program called TIPS is training ordinary people specifically to prevent drunk driving. The TIPS program (Training for Intervention Procedures by Servers of Alcohol) gives people—parents, students, bartenders, vendors, teachers, waiters, store clerks, and the like—the skills and confidence to intervene when they recognize patterns of alcohol abuse.

TIPS has been proven highly effective by independent studies, and has been embraced by the hospitality and insurance industries. It has won numerous awards, including the National Commission Against

Drunk Driving's Education and Prevention Award, and has been recognized by the Department of Transportation for saving lives and changing behavior. President George Bush recommended that everyone be TIPS trained.

TIPS-trained bar personnel not only help people to enjoy alcohol but also prevent people from abusing alcohol and prevent drunk driving. To date, TIPS has trained almost 500,000 people in twenty countries.

Chapter 16

Prevention

If we could discover the early warning signs of cancer, perhaps 95 percent of incipient cancers could be arrested. We already know the early warning signs of alcohol problems.

How can alcoholism be prevented?

Alcoholism will never be prevented by a simple vaccine or a magic formula. It doesn't have a single cause, so it will not have a single cure or a single preventive treatment.

The early warning signs of alcoholism are already known, the trick is making them work. I believe society should take two major steps to prevent alcoholism, as I define it. These steps would make it easier to recognize people who are using alcohol poorly and to offer help before alcohol problems develop. First, a consensus on guidelines should be established on **How to Drink, Where to Drink, When to Drink,** and **How Much to Drink.** When practical guidelines are established as the norm for social drinking, people will be less likely to solve their problems with alcohol.

This consensus on guidelines would require a profound change in attitude and behavior, and I believe it could be accomplished through enlightened education, inspired national leadership, and concerned community organization. If you doubt the potential for change in society, recall how fifty years ago a famous movie star's career was destroyed when she conceived a child out of wedlock, or that a short time ago coed dorms were inconceivable. Compare the public reaction then with today's laissez-faire attitude. Change happens. Why? Because society can and does set new standards.

A sound consensus on guidelines would set the stage for the second step in prevention. The second step would establish methods for people to help one another. One such method has already been established: the TIPS program. (See below)

The truism of all health and social issues would operate: The earlier a problem is diagnosed and treated, the better the solution and the lower the cost.

I enjoy drinking, and I don't want to quit. How can I be sure I won't become an alcoholic?

You can be sure that you won't become an alcoholic, up to a point, by following the guidelines of safe drinking given earlier in Chapter 3, and by paying attention to the purpose and pattern of your drinking.

You say you enjoy drinking. Ask yourself, what does alcohol do for you? Is your response bizarre or unusual? Do you *need* alcohol to function? Look closely, heed what you see, and if a problem is developing, you can do something about it.

Has prohibition of alcohol ever succeeded?

Even under totalitarian regimes, attempts at prohibition have failed. The Koran forbids drinking, and yet Pan-Arabic Alcoholism Conferences are held annually. At an international meeting of world prohibitionists in Kabul, Afganistan, I once met a gentleman from a small state in India who assured me that prohibition was working in his state. I didn't dispute him, but it would be a first.

What is society's role in prevention?

Society's role in prevention is a subject so complex and of such broad implications that it demands a book of its own, and goes beyond the purpose of this one. Indeed, a truly effective national approach to prevention goes far beyond education, information pamphlets, and clever slogans. It requires that people examine their national values and, in some instances, alter their social environment.

Society needs to consider ways that business and industry can alleviate the anxiety of their employees and to help workers see the worth of their individual contributions.

In moving to a deeper level, does the insatiable national striving for bigness create a tense and worried population? What can we do about it as individuals or as part of a group? For instance, what are we teaching our children about alcohol by *our* example?

The questions are difficult, the list is long, but Americans can and have made many beneficial changes in their lives, and I believe that they can do it again. The bits and pieces of change brought about by individual and community action are powerful, but they must be based on understanding and caring about human needs; such endeavors can prevent alcohol abuse.

A program for prevention that works: TIPS

The TIPS program was specifically designed to prevent drunk driving. The program's remarkable thrust uses the powerful preventive impact of one person trained to help another. Education frees the mind from the shackles of ignorance, and TIPS provides both the education and the skills to empower the person with the confidence to take action and intervene.

The TIPS programs were created not only for sellers and servers of alcohol, i.e., personnel in restaurants, bars, hotels, stadiums, convenience stores, and social functions, but also for parents, universities, and the workplace. TIPS is known as the CPR and Heimlich method of alcohol abuse.

Epilogue

If I said to you simply, I drink, you might well think to yourself: What a shame. Such a nice man. How his family must suffer! Then I might add that not only do I drink but so do my wife and children and, occasionally, my grandchildren.

I received my first taste of alcohol at my ritual circumcision when I was eight days old. Alcohol was part of my family and social life. It was part of my life at college and medical school. Alcohol was neither prohibited nor recognized as something to be avoided or sought after. It was just there. I considered it as just one of the many gifts of life—to use at my discretion. I suppose I could have focused on the negatives, of which there were plenty, but I focused on the pleasures, of which there were many.

I guess my attitude toward drinking alcohol stems from my philosphical bent to look for the pony in the dung—to see the glass as half full, not half empty. I decided early on that I was going to enjoy life and its pleasures.

I'm not talking about the pleasures of the body

alone, but all pleasures. I like the bite of cold, clear air in my lungs as I stand alone with my skis on top of a mountain. I find pleasure in wandering through ancient ruins and visiting foreign cities, in watching the clouds pass by in the sky, in observing the spectacular show of autumn leaves. I thrill to the sound of music, to the sound of laughing children, to all the noises that tell me I'm alive.

And it is true that the pursuit of a full life is frought with vagaries and unmet expectations. Astonishingly, there are some people who are afraid of life and uncomfortable with pleasure. When they do permit themselves to drink, for example, it is often done abusively.

Readers of this book do not abuse alcohol and know that drinking enhances and embellishes the gifts of life. No words I can offer will recall the immediate pleasure, sight, taste, and smell of wine, for example. Some forms of alcohol will fade quickly from the palate's memory like a passing acquaintance, while others will linger forever like a true friend.

Now that we have reached this point of our penetrating look at alcohol, what do we see? No one questions the popularity of alcohol throughout the world, and here at home. The book's exposition of the time-tested popularity of alcohol seems reasonable, considering the evidence and arguments—both historical and technical.

And anyone who has confidence in the intelligence and endurance of the human race will not worry that another prohibition will be any different from the march of prohibitions that have peppered our history. When that characteristically prescient property of *We the People* decides that too much drinking is creating conditions that run counter to its interests, alcohol consumption will decline.

We do have a few measuring rods that enable people to gauge their drinking patterns. For instance, if you answer yes to any of the following questions, you're in trouble. Do you drink more than others in your group? Are you always pressing for the next round? Do you lie about how much you drink? Are your work and family life being crowded out of first place? Do you lose interest in food when drinking?

A good night's sleep represents the end of a drinking occasion for social drinkers. For the problem drinker, however, it means a long period of abstinence. The point of the proof is that alcohol for the problem drinker has become essential. Within social drinking practices, the definition of moderation is of no great matter. Most people have figured out their drinking habits.

There is indeed amusement in the extremes. Nearly all of us knows the person who thinks "bad" once a year on New Year's Eve after a glass of elderberry wine. Just up on another rung are those who think they'd better be on guard because hardly a week has gone by for months when they did not take a drink.

On the other hand, we have the immortal words

of William Shakespeare who proclaimed: "Ale is a dish for a king." And we're emboldened by the stirring words of Thomas Jefferson, who understood the fragility of people when he guaranteed our "unalienable rights . . . life, liberty, and the pursuit of happiness." Robert Burns, with staid but sensible advice, pointed out that "a man may drink and not be drunk." Charles Dickens, whose novels are remarkable for their rich portraits of society and their crusades against abuses, described the tone of his times: "Fan the sinking flame of hilarity with the wing of friendship; and pass the rosy wine."

How much is too much is no longer anyone's guess. Queen Victoria was accustomed to taking a daily dram in her tea. If you are near the center and between the extremes, you probably have heretofore given the matter little thought, but now you know that individual tolerance, personality, expectations, settings, and body weight do matter and add to our understanding. One person with the same blood-alcohol level may seem to be unaffected and another sloppily tipsy. One may be quiet and morose and the other entirely too boisterous.

With some assurance we can say that alcohol is a substance that can kill you quickly and surely, but no more quickly or surely than water, if you drink too much of it at one time. Alcohol is actually manufactured in the body but is less damaging than other natural secretions from glands such as the thyroid, pituitary, adrenal, and pancreas. Alcohol in moderate amounts is not only harmless to the body but also beneficial in many cases.

Alcohol is a valuable substance. As a sedative and a food, it can be used for these properties in many conditions. In addition, alcohol can stimulate a flagging appetite and generate interest in social interaction for the aged or chronically ill people.

In moderate amounts alcohol and sex have synergistic benefits; in heavy amounts alcohol prevents performance.

In the history of the human race, alcohol has a conspicuous position. It can trace its lineage to religion, science and agriculture, it enhances confidence and promotes goodwill. It is an efficient and practical relaxer for the driving force in the brain; it offers immediate personal enjoyment; it is a social lubricant. And it enables us to forget, at least for a little while, the shortness of life and the ludicrously helpless and infinitesimally small part we play in the history of the universe.

Moderate alcohol use is neither unhealthy nor dangerous. The danger lies in overindulgence.

Alcohol use has always accommodated the conventions of a given culture in any given time. Today the average drinker balances restraint with relaxation within his or her own personal capacity.

And finally, we can say that alcohol has existed longer than recorded history. It has outlived generations, nations, epochs, and ages. It is a part of us, and that is our good fortune.

Index

AA. *See* Alcoholics Anonymous

abuse. *See* alcohol abuse; drug abuse

addiction: to alcohol, 47–48; definition of, 38

addictive personality, 38–39

adolescence. *See* drinking, teenagers

Aeschylus, 15

alcohol: acculturation of, 86; addiction to, 47–48; calories, 45, 52; content in drinks, 48–49; denatured, 49; for digestion, 67; drug interactions, 77–83; facts about, 43–50; and feelings, 73–75; and health, 63–71; history of, 15–24; how it makes you high, 50; how to keep from overreacting to, 27; as hunger suppressant, 45–46; as medication, 66; national consumption, 74; negative preoccupation with, 9–13; persistent notions about, 31–42; pharmacologic action of, 43–44; physical effects, 25, 46, 51–58; rubbing, 50; and sleep, 68; and social interaction, 85–90; strength in drinks, 49; use of, 3, 11; value

of, 127; worldwide sales, 93. *See also* drinking

alcohol abuse, 3, 85–86; prevention of, 117–21; problem of, 9–13

alcoholics: children of, 4, 32, 107; hidden, 4; nondrinking, 12; recovering, 35–36; women, 33–34

Alcoholics Anonymous (AA), 52, 96

alcohol interactions: antibiotics, 79; anticoagulants, 79; anticonvulsants, 80; antidepressants, 80; antidiabetics, 82; antihistamines, 78, 82; antipsychotics, 82; barbiturates, 78, 81; benzodiazepines, 80–81; calcium channel blockers, 81; diuretics, 83; hypnotics, 80–81; nonsteroidal anti-inflammatory drugs (NSAIDs), 80; opioids, 82; sedatives, 78, 80–81; sleeping pills, 80–81

alcoholism, 58; cure for, 34–35; disease of, 32; ethnicity and, 96; hereditary, 32–33; in medicine, 98–99; prevention of, 117–18,

118–19; rates of, 94–95; withdrawal symptoms, 56
American history: alcohol and, 20–24
Anstie, Francis, 26
Anstie's Law of Safe Drinking, 26
Antabuse (disulfiram), 82–83
antialcoholics: alcohol interactions, 82–83
aperitifs, 19
aphrodisiac: alcohol as, 31
appetite: alcohol and, 45–46, 66–67
Aristotle, 15
arteries: hardening of, 42
aspirin, 78

BAC (blood-alcohol concentration), 112
barbiturates, alcohol interactions, 78, 81
bars: what they can do about drunk driving, 114–15
bed spins, after drinking, 57–58
beer: alcohol content, 48–49; for digestion, 67; mixing with liquor, 41
beer belly: causes of, 54
behavior. *See* drinking behavior
benzodiazepines, alcohol interactions, 80–81
Bible: wine in, 17–18, 86
body weight: and drinking, 44–45, 51–52
boiler-makers, 41
brain: alcohol and, 39–40, 65
Breathalyzer, 112–13
Bush, George, 115
business: alcohol in, 97–98

calcium channel blockers, alcohol interactions, 81

California: vineyards, 20
calories: in alcohol, 45, 52
Canada: drinking age, 108
carbonated mixers, 62
children: of alcoholics, 4, 32, 107; drinking patterns, 103–109; what to teach, 105–107
China: drinking in, 15, 28
Churchill, Winston, 9, 12
cirrhosis, 70
cocaine, alcohol interactions, 81–82
coffee: to sober up, 40
cold showers: to sober up, 40
Cortez, 20

demon rum, 22
denatured alcohol, 49
dependent personalities, 4
depression: with drinking, 73–74
diet: drinking man's, 52–53
digestion: alcohol and, 67
distilled alcohol, 18–19
diuretics, alcohol interactions, 83
drinking: best of, 25–30; business advantages, 101; expectations, 88; group, 86–87; guidelines for, 26–30; how, 26–27; how much, 26; moderately, 6, 10, 63–64, 126–27; peer pressure, 89; physical effects, 56–57; responsible, 30; safe, 26–30, 111; social, 51; teenage, 103–104, 104–105, 107–108, 109; thirst with, 55–56; two-fisted, 6; U.S. heritage, 91–96; when, 27–28; where, 28–29. *See also* heavy drinking; problem drinking
drinking age, 108
drinking behavior, 91; influence of

New World on, 22–23; learned, 107

drinking companions, 29–30

drinking habits, values and, 91, 96

drinking sprees: health hazards, 70

drinks: alcohol contents, 48–49; alcohol strength, 49; diluting, 46–47; need for, 74–75; switching, 62. *See also* beer; wine; liquors

driving: alcohol-related accidents, 113; drinking and, 111–15; impaired, 112. *See also* drunk driving

drug abuse, 10–11

drugs: alcohol interactions, 77–83; definition of, 11; that are dangerous with alcohol, 78–79. *See also* alcoholic interactions

drunk driving, 111; what bars can do about, 114–15; what you can do about, 113–14

drunkenness: preventing, 39

dry mouth, 67

education: about drinking, 105–107

Egypt: history of wine in, 15

elderly: alcohol for, 65–66

Ericson, Leif, 20

ethnicity: and alcoholism, 96

ethyl alcohol, 15

feelings: alcohol and, 73–75

food: alcohol absorption and, 47

Food and Drug Administration, definition of drug, 11

fools: at parties, 88

France: alcohol problems, 91–92, 95; vineyards, 18, 20. *See also* vineyards

Franciscans, 20

friendliness: drinking and, 87

"Friends don't let friends drive drunk," 114

Germany, vineyards, 20

Greece, history of wine in, 15–16

group drinking, 86–87

Ham, 17

hangovers, 59–62; conditions that predispose to, 60; cures, 62; definition of, 59; how to avoid, 61, 62; how to kill, 37–38, 40; how to treat, 61; reasons for, 60

health: alcohol and, 63–71; drinking spree hazards, 70

heart: effects of alcohol on, 64–65

heavy drinkers: associating with, 36–37; when they stop drinking, 56

heavy drinking, 58; adverse physical effects of, 70–71; and nutrition, 69

high: how alcohol makes you feel, 50

history: of alcohol, 15–24; alcohol's role in, 19–20. *See also* history of wine

homemakers: with drinking problems, 100

hooliganism, 109

hunger suppressant, alcohol as, 45–46

hypnotics, alcohol interactions, 80–81

hypotension: postural, 58

inhibition: and alcohol, 73

intelligence: alcohol and, 39–40

intimacy: drinking and, 75

Irish: rate of alcoholism, 94–95
isopropyl, 50
Italy: alcohol problems, 95; history
    of wine in, 16; vineyards, 20.
    See also vineyards

Japan: drinking habits, 93–94
Jerusalem: history of wine in, 15
Jesuits, 20
Jesus, 18
job: drinking on the, 97–101

kidney disease: alcohol and, 41–42
Koran, 119; wine making in, 17–18

legal intoxication, 112
"Liquor after beer, never fear; beer
    after liquor, never sicker," 41
liquors: alcohol contents, 48–49;
    diluting, 46–47; rum, 21–22;
    whiskey, 19, 22, 41
liver. *See* cirrhosis of
long life: moderate drinking and,
    63–64
low blood pressure, 58

marijuana (cannabis): alcohol in-
    teractions, 81–82
Marlboro Man, 30
medication: alcohol as, 66. *See
    also* drugs
medicine, alcoholism in, 98–99
military: drinking problems in, 98
milk: to prevent drunkenness, 39
mixers: carbonated, 62
moderate drinking, 6, 10, 126–27;
    and long life, 63–64

NASA, 62
Nation, Carry, 9, 12
nations: problem-drinking, 91–92

Native Americans: rate of alcohol-
    ism, 94–95
New England: rum in, 21–22
New World: influence on drinking
    behavior, 22–23
Noah, 17
nonsteroidal anti-inflammatory
    drugs (NSAIDs), alcohol inter-
    actions, 80
NSAID. *See* nonsteroidal anti-in-
    flammatory drugs
nutrition: drinking and, 68–69

occupational drinking, 97–101
opioids, alcohol interactions, 82

Pan-Arabic Alcoholism Confer-
    ences, 119
parties, 87–88; cocktail, 28–29,
    88–89
peer pressure, 89
Persian folklore, history of wine in,
    16
pharmacology: of alcohol, 43–44
Plato, 15
Poe, Edgar Allan, 99
poison: alcohol as, 16–17
polydipsia, 51
postural hypotension, 58
power people: with drinking prob-
    lems, 99
preoccupation: problem of, 9–13
prevention, 39, 117–21; society's
    role in, 119–20; TIPS program,
    120–21
problem drinking, 4; among teen-
    agers, 108, 109; *vs* social drink-
    ing, 11
professions: with high rates of al-
    coholism, 98–99, 100–101
prohibition, 23, 119; historical fail-

ure of, 4–5; logic underlying, 35; present wave, 23–24
Prozac (fluoxetine), 80
Puritans, 21

recovering alcoholics, 35–36
red noses: causes of, 54–55
red wine, 20; *vs* white wine, 40–41
relationships, 85–86
relaxation: with alcohol, 73
religious affiliation: and drinking, 89–90
ritual services: alcohol in, 18, 86
Romans: history of wine in, 16
rubbing alcohol, 50
rum, 21–22; alcohol content, 48–49
Russia: drinking problems, 91–92, 109

safe drinking, 111; Anstie's Law of, 26; guidelines for, 26–30
salicylate drugs, 78
Sappho, 15
Satan, 17
sedatives, alcohol interactions and, 78, 80–81
sex lives: of drinkers, 53–54
showers: to sober up, 40
Skid Row, 53, 87
slave trade: association with rum, 22
sleep, effects of alcohol on, 68
sleeping pills: alcohol interactions and, 80–81
social drinking, 51; *vs* problem drinking, 11
social interaction: alcohol and, 85–90
society: role in prevention, 119–20. *See* prevention

Socrates, 15, 104–105
Spain, vineyards, 20
spirits: alcohol content, 48–49; diluting, 46–47
sports: alcohol problems in, 99
spouses of famous people: with drinking problems, 99–100
straight alcohol: birth of, 18–19
Sweden, drinking problems, 91–92, 109
switching drinks, 62

teenage drinking. *See* drinking
Theologicum, 18
thirst: with drinking, 55–56
threshold resistances, 65
TIPS (Training for Intervention Procedures by Servers of Alcohol) program, 111, 114–15, 118, 120–21
tipsiness: after drinking, 58
two-drink person, 6
two-fisted drinking, 6
Tylenol (acetaminophen), 78

ulcers: drinking with, 67–68
United States: alcohol consumption, 74; alcohol history, 20–24; alcohol problems, 91–92, 96; alcohol-related driving accidents, 113; drinking age, 108; drinking heritage, 91–96; drinking patterns, 91, 92–93
United States Congress: alcoholism in, 99
urine tests, 112–13
U.S. Constitution: Eighteenth Amendment, 5, 23

values, drinking habits and, 91, 96
Victoria, 126

vineyards, 18, 20
Vinland, 20
viticulture: history of, 15–18, 20

Washington, D.C.: drinking pattern, 92–93
weight gain: when you stop drinking, 51–52
whiskey, 19; American production of, 22; beer chasers, 41

white wine, 20; *vs* red wine, 40–41
wine, 86; alcohol content, 48–49; for digestion, 67; history of, 15–18; red, 20, 40–41; white, 20, 40–41
Wineland, 20
withdrawal, 56
women: alcoholics, 33–34
work, drinking at, 97–101
writers: with alcohol problems, 99

About The Authors

Morris E. Chafetz, M.D., is widely recognized as one of the world's foremost authorities on alcohol use and abuse. He is the founding director of the National Institute on Alcohol Abuse and Alcoholism (NIAAA) in the U.S. Department of Health and Human Services. During his tenure at NIAAA, Dr. Chafetz was pivotal in removing the stigma from alcoholic people. Prior to his government service, Dr. Chafetz served as associate clinical professor of psychiatry at Harvard Medical School, director of clinical psychiatric services, and chief of the Alcohol Clinic at the Massachusetts General Hospital in Boston.

President Reagan appointed Dr. Chafetz to the Presidential Commission on Drunk Driving as chairman of the Committee on Education and Prevention. Today he serves on the Board of Directors and on the Communications Committee of the National Commission Against Drunk Driving.

Dr. Chafetz is president and founder of the Health Education Foundation, an organization that relates health to lifestyle. The foundation is responsible for creating TIPS (Training for Intervention Procedures by Servers of Alcohol), a skills-training program designed to prevent alcohol abuse.

Dr. Chafetz has written and collaborated on two hundred scientific and popular articles and fourteen books, including *Alcoholism and Society*; *Frontiers of Alcoholism*; *Why Drinking Can Be Good for You*; *Youth, Alcohol and Social Policy*; *The Encyclopedia of Alcoholism*; and *The Alcoholic Patient: Diagnosis and Management*. He writes for the Encyclopedia Britannica's *Medical and Health Annual* on alcohol abuse and alcoholism and reviews books for the *New England Journal of Medicine*. His most recent book, *Obsession: The Bizarre Relationship Between a Prominent Harvard Psychiatrist and Her Suicidal Patient*, was coauthored with son Gary Chafetz.

Marion D. Chafetz is editor in chief of publications at the Health Education Foundation, a nonprofit organization that designs health promotion programs, publishes books and pamphlets, and distributes a quarterly newsletter on health issues.

She has traveled extensively for thirty years to most parts of the world with her husband, Dr. Chafetz, collecting data on alcohol problems and programs. For the past fifteen years Mrs. Chafetz has edited professional articles and books on alcohol use and abuse and has coauthored an annual update on alcohol and alcoholism for the Encyclopedia Britannica.

Mrs. Chafetz served as a staff member to Nelson

Rockefeller's National Commission on Water Quality. She was responsible for the study and synopsis of EPA development documents and strategy papers, the analysis of contractors studies for commission members, and the classification of technical and professional comments for commission reports.

As board member of the D.C. Health Planning Advisory Commission, she advised the mayor on the health needs of the District of Columbia.

Mrs. Chafetz has written numerous health publications including *Health Education: An Annotated Bibliography of Lifestyle, Behavior and Health*; *HEF NEWS*; *Health Fact Tips*; and *Minding Your Mind*.